About the Author

Dr. B.S. Dhillon is a professor of Mechanical Engineering at the University of Ottawa. He has served as a Chairman/Director of Mechanical Engineering Department/Engineering Management Program for over 10 years at the same institution. He has published over 300 articles on reliability, safety, maintainability, etc. He is or has been on the editorial boards of 7 international scientific journals. In addition, Dr. Dhillon has written 25 books on various aspects of human factors, reliability, safety, maintainability, and design published by Wiley (1981), Van Nostrand (1982), Butterworth (1983), Marcel Dekker (1984), Pergamon (1986), McGraw-Hill (1996), etc. In 1986, he wrote the first ever book on human reliability (published by the Pergamon Press) and in 2000, he wrote the second ever book on medical device reliability (published by the CRC Press). His books on reliability have been translated into many languages including Russian, Chinese and German. He has served as General Chairman of two international conferences on reliability and quality control held in Los Angeles and Paris in 1987.

Dr. Dhillon is recipient of the American Society of Quality Control Austin J. Bonis Reliability Award, the Society of Reliability Engineers' Merit Award, the Gold Medal of Honor (American Biographical Institute), and the Faculty of Engineering Glinski Award for Excellence in Research. He is a registered Professional Engineer in Ontario and is listed in the American Men and Women of Science, Men of Achievements, International Dictionary of Biography, Who's Who in International Intellectuals, and Who's Who in Technology.

Dr. Dhillon has served as a consultant to various organizations and bodies (including the Ottawa Heart Institute and the World Heart Corporation) and has many years of experience in the industrial sector. At the University of Ottawa, he has been teaching reliability, maintainability, safety, and other related areas for over 23 years and he has also lectured in over 50 countries. Professor Dhillon attended the University of Wales where he received a BS in electrical and electronic engineering and an MS in mechanical engineering. He received a PhD in industrial engineering from the University of Windsor.

SERIES ON INDUSTRIAL AND SYSTEMS ENGINEERING

Series Editor: Hoang Pham (*Rutgers University*)

Series on Industrial & Systems Engineering – Vol. 2

Human Reliability and Error in Medical System

B. S. Dhillon

University of Ottawa, Canada

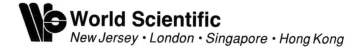
World Scientific
New Jersey · London · Singapore · Hong Kong

Published by

World Scientific Publishing Co. Pte. Ltd.

5 Toh Tuck Link, Singapore 596224

USA office: Suite 202, 1060 Main Street, River Edge, NJ 07661

UK office: 57 Shelton Street, Covent Garden, London WC2H 9HE

Library of Congress Cataloging-in-Publication Data
Dhillon, B. S.
    Human reliability and error in medical system / B.S. Dhillon.
       p. cm. -- (Series on industrial and system engineering ; . 2)
    Includes bibliographical references and index.
    ISBN 981-238-359-X
    1. Biomedical engineering. 2. Human engineering. 3. Reliability (Engineering). I. Title.
    II. Series.

    R855.3.D467 2003
    610'.28--dc21   2003053538

British Library Cataloguing-in-Publication Data
A catalogue record for this book is available from the British Library.

Desk Editor: Tjan Kwang Wei

Printed in Singapore by World Scientific Printers (S) Pte Ltd

This book is affectionately dedicated to the memory of my late PhD dissertation supervisor Professor Charles L. Proctor.

Contents

Preface

Human reliability and error have become a very important issue in health care due to the occurrence of a vast number of associated deaths each year, particularly, in nations where equality creates inequality. For example, as indicated in the findings of the Institute of Medicine in 1999, around 100000 Americans die due to human error each year. This means human error in health care is the 8th leading cause of death in the United States. More specifically, the number of people who died due to human error in health care is equivalent to the combined figure for deaths due to motor vehicle accidents (43500), breast cancer (42300), and AIDS (16500) in a given year. Moreover, the total annual national cost resulting from the medical errors is estimated to be between US $17 billion and US $29 billion.

Although, the history of human reliability may be traced back to 1958, the commencement of serious thoughts on human reliability or human error in medical system dates back only to the period around the late 1970s. Since the 1970s over 500 journal and conference proceedings publications on human reliability or error in medicine have appeared. As increasing attention is being paid to human error in health care the need for a book covering the basics and essentials of general human reliability, errors, and human factors as well as the comprehensive and latest information on human reliability and error in medical system is considered absolutely necessary.

Currently, such information is either available in specialized articles or books, but not in a single volume. This causes a great deal of difficulty to information seekers since they have to consult many different and diverse sources.

This book is written to satisfy this vital need. The sources of the material presented is given in the references at the end of each chapter. This will be useful to readers if they desire to delve deeper into a particular area. The book contains a chapter on mathematical concepts necessary to understand materials presented in subsequent chapters. However, the other topics covered in the volume are treated in such a manner that the reader will require no previous knowledge to understand its contents. At appropriate places, the book contains examples along with their solutions and at the end of each chapter there are numerous problems to test the reader's comprehension in the subject. A comprehensive list of references on human error and reliability in health care is provided at the end of the book to give readers a view of the intensity of developments in the field.

The book is composed of eleven chapters. Chapter 1 presents the various introductory aspects of human reliability and error in medical system including medical-error-related facts and figures, terms and definitions, as well as other useful information. Chapter 2 is devoted to mathematical concepts useful for performing the analysis of human reliability and error in health care and it covers topics such as the Boolean algebra laws, probability distributions, Laplace transforms, and first order differential equations.

Chapter 3 presents the human factors basics including human behaviors, human sensory capacities, human body measurements, and human factors-related formulas and data sources. Human reliability and error basics are presented in Chapter 4. It covers topics such as human performance reliability and correctability functions, human reliability analysis methods, reasons for human error occurrence, and human error analysis models.

Chapter 5 presents a total of nine methods extracted from published literature considered useful for performing human reliability and error analysis in health care. These methods include failure modes and effect analysis (FMEA), root cause analysis (RCA), cause and effect diagram, Markov method, hazard and operability study (HAZOP), and fault tree analysis (FTA).

Chapters 6 and 7 are devoted to human error in medication and anesthesia, respectively. Some of the topics covered in Chapter 6 are medication error facts and figures, types and causes of medication errors, medication errors in hospitals, medication error reduction, and medication-error-related studies. Chapter 7 includes topics such as anesthesia-related facts and figures, frequent anesthesia errors, methods for preventing anesthetic mishaps, and anesthesia error-related studies.

Chapter 8 presents human error in miscellaneous health care areas and health care human error cost. Some of the specific topics covered are human error in intensive care units, emergency medicine, operating rooms, and laboratory testing; and health-care human error-related cost studies and cost estimation models.

Chapter 9 presents the various important areas of human factors in medical devices including related facts and figures, human error causing use interface design problems, an approach to human factors in the development process of medical devices, rules of thumb for device control/display arrangement and design, installation, software design, and alarms with respect to users, as well as human error analysis methods for medical devices.

Chapters 10 and 11 are devoted to mathematical models for predicting human reliability and error in the medical systems as well as health care human error reporting systems and data, respectively. Some of the topics covered in Chapter 10 are mathematical models for determining human performance reliability in normal environment, in alternating environment, and with critical and non-critical errors, and human correctability function. Chapter 11 includes topics such as the review of current human error-related health care reporting systems, lessons from non-medical near miss reporting systems, state adverse medical event reporting systems, and medical human error-related data sources.

This book will be useful to many individuals including health care professionals, administrators, and students, human factors/psychology specialists, health care researchers and instructors, biomedical engineers, safety professionals, and graduate students in biomedical engineering.

The author is deeply indebted to many individuals including students, colleagues, and friends for their invisible inputs and encouragement in moments of need. I thank my children Jasmine and Mark for their patience and intermittent disturbances leading to desirable coffee and other breaks. Last, but not least, I thank my other half, friend, and wife, Rosy, for typing various portions of this book and other related materials, and for her timely help in proofreading.

B.S. Dhillon
Ottawa, Ontario

Chapter 1

Introduction

1.1 Background

Medicine has been identified as a profession for the past 3000 years and today a vast sum of money is spent on health care worldwide.[1] For example, in 1997, the world market for medical devices alone was estimated to be around $120 billion.[2] Humans (i.e. doctors, nurses, etc.) are a critical component of the health care system and they are subjected to errors.

Nonetheless, it may be added that human error is a fact of life. More specifically, it occurs in all aspects of life and in every job occupation with varying consequences. In addition, as in Ref. 3, an average of 60–80% of all accidents involve human error in one way or the other. Although the occurrence of human error in medicine may have been there ever since its first practice, the earliest documented medical error-related death in modern times may be traced back to 1848.[4,5] It was associated with the administering of anesthetic.

It appears that the first serious studies concerned with medical errors were conducted in the late 1950s and the early 1960s,[6,7] mainly focusing on anesthesia-related deaths. Since the early 1960s, a large number of publications on human error in medical system have appeared, and a comprehensive list of these publications is provided in the appendix.

1.2 Medical Error-Related Facts and Figures

This section presents the facts and figures directly or indirectly related to the subject of human error in the health care system.

- In a typical year around 100000 Americans die due to human errors.[8] The financial impact of these errors on the US economy is estimated to be somewhere between $17 billion and $29 billion.[8]
- Operator errors account for more than 50% of all technical medical equipment problems.[9]
- A study of anesthetic incidents in operating rooms revealed that between 70% and 82% of the incidents were due to human errors.[10,11]
- Human error accounts for 60% of all medical device-related deaths or injuries reported through the Center for Devices and Radiological Health (CDRH) of the Food and Drug Administration (FDA).[12]
- In 1993, a total of 7391 people died due to medication errors in the United States alone.[8,13]
- The annual cost of medication errors is estimated to be over $7 billion in the United States.[14]
- In the interpretation of radiographs, the rates of disagreement between emergency physicians and radiologists vary from 8–11%.[15]
- In the emergency departments over 90% of the adverse events are considered preventable.[16]
- A study revealed that the annual avoidable deaths from anesthesia-associated incidents hovered between 2000 and 10000 in the United States.[17,18]
- A study of critical incident reports, in an intensive care unit, over a ten year period (i.e. from 1989–1999) revealed that most of the incidents were due to staff errors and not equipment failures.[19]
- An examination of 14 Australian studies published during the period between 1988 and 1996 revealed that 2.4 to 3.6% of all hospital admissions were drug-related and approximately 32–69% were preventable.[20]
- In the United States, the annual cost of hospital-based medication-related errors is estimated to be around $2 billion.[21]
- Medication errors exist between 5.3% and 20.6% of all administered doses.[22]
- A major Hong Kong teaching hospital administered 16000 anesthetics in one year and reported 125 related critical incidents, in which human error was an important factor (i.e. in 80% of the cases).[23]
- In 1984, a study examined the records of 2.7 million patients discharged from hospitals in New York and it was found that 25% of the 98609 patients who suffered from an adverse event was the result of negligence.[24]
- An investigation of 5612 surgical admissions to a hospital revealed a total of 36 adverse outcomes due to human error.[25]

- In 589 anesthesia-related deaths, human error was considered to be a factor in 83% of the cases.[6,26]
- During the period between 1970 and 1977, a total of 277 anesthetic-related deaths occurred and factors such as faulty technique (43%), coexistent disease (12%), failure of postoperative care (10%), and drug overdose (5%) were considered to be responsible for the deaths.[27]

1.3 Terms and Definitions

This section presents some useful terms and definitions, whether directly or indirectly, related to human reliability/error in health care.[8,28–32]

- **Human error.** This refers to the failure to perform a given task (or the performance of a forbidden action) that could result in the disruption of scheduled operations or damage to property and equipment.
- **Human reliability.** This refers to the probability of performing a task successfully by humans at any required stage in a system operation within a specified minimum time limit (if the time requirement is specified).
- **Medical technology.** This is the equipment, drugs, procedures, and the methods used by professionals working in health care institutions to deliver medical care to people. This term includes the systems within which such care is delivered.
- **Risk.** This refers to the probable rate of occurrence of a hazardous situation as well as the degree of the harm severity.
- **Accident.** This is an event that involves damage to a specified system that suddenly disrupts the ongoing or potential output of the system.
- **Adverse event.** This is an injury due to a medical intervention.
- **Human factors.** This is a study of the interrelationships between humans, the tools they employ or use, and the surrounding environment in which they work and live.
- **Continuous task.** This is a task that involves some kind of tracking activity (e.g. monitoring a changing situation).
- **Human performance.** This is a measure of failures and actions under specified conditions.
- **Human performance reliability.** This refers to the probability that a human will successfully perform all required functions subjected to specified conditions.
- **Health care organization.** This is an entity that provides, coordinates, and/or insures medical-related services for the public/people.

- **Anesthesiology.** This is a branch of the medical field that deals with the processes of rendering patients insensitive to various types of pain during surgery or when faced with chronic/acute pain states.
- **Medication error.** This refers to any preventable events that may cause or result in wrong medication use or patient harm while the medication is in the control of a patient, a consumer, or a health care professional.
- **Patient safety.** This is the freedom from accidental injury. Ensuring patient safety involves the creation of operational systems/processes that reduce the likelihood of error occurrence.
- **Fault.** This is an immediate cause of a failure.
- **Failure.** This is the inability of an item to carry out its specified function.
- **Failure mode.** This is the consequence of the mechanism through which the failure in question occurs.
- **Operator error.** This is an error that occurs when an item operator does not adhere to the correct procedures.
- **Mission time.** This is that element of uptime needed to carry out a specified mission profile.
- **Consequence.** This is an outcome of an accident (e.g. human fatalities, environmental pollution, and damage to properties).
- **Hazardous situation.** This is a condition with a potential to threaten human life, health, properties, or the environment.
- **Human error consequence.** This is an undesired consequence of human failure/error.

1.4   Useful Information on Human Reliability and Error in Medicine

This section lists down some of the books, journals, conference proceedings, and organizations which are useful in obtaining information on human reliability and error in health care related issues.

1.4.1   *Books*

Some of the books that focus on human error in health care are listed here as follows:

- Bogner, M.S. (ed), *Human Error in Medicine*, Lawrence Erlbaum Associates, Publishers, Hillsdale, New Jersey, 1994.

- Spath, P.L. (ed), *Error Reduction in Health Care*, Jossey-Bass Publications, San Francisco, California, 1999.
- Kohn, L.T., Corrigan, J.M. and Donaldson, M.S. (eds), *To Err is Human: Building a Safer Health System*, National Academy Press, Washington, D.C., 1999.
- Rosenthal, M.M. and Sutcliffe, K.M. (eds), *Medical Error: What Do We Know? What Do We Do?*, John Wiley and Sons, New York, 2002.
- Mulcahy, L., Lloyd-Bostock, S.M. and Rosenthal, M.M., *Medical Mishaps: Pieces of the Puzzle*, Taylor and Francis, Inc., New York, 1999.
- Caldwell, C. and Denham, C., *Reducing Medication Errors and Recovering Costs: A Four-Step Approach for Executives*, Health Administration Press, Chicago, 2001.
- Cohen, J., *ER: Enter at Your Own Risk: How to Avoid Dangers inside Emergency Rooms*, New Horizon Press, Far Hills, New Jersey, 2001.
- Mociver, S., *Medical Nightmares: The Human Face of Errors*, Chestnut Publishing Group, Toronto, Canada, 2002.
- Youngson, R.M. and Schott, I., *Medical Blunders: Amazing True Stories of Mad, Bad, and Dangerous Doctors*, New York University Press, New York, 1996.
- Dhillon, B.S., *Medical Device Reliability: and Associated Areas*, CRC Press, Boca Raton, Florida, 2000, Chapter 4.

1.4.2 *Journals*

The scientific journals that contain articles directly or indirectly related to human error in medicine are as follows:

- New England Journal of Medicine
- American Family Physician
- Anesthesia
- British Journal of Anesthesia
- Canadian Journal of Anesthesia
- British Medical Journal
- Canadian Medical Association Journal
- European Journal of Anesthesiology
- Journal of Clinical Anesthesia
- Journal of American Medical Association (JAMA)
- Journal of Family Practice
- Journal of General Internal Medicine

- Journal of Nursing Administration
- Journal of Professional Nursing
- Journal of Quality Clinical Practice
- Journal of Royal Society of Medicine
- Journal of the American College of Surgeons
- Medical Device Diagnostic Industry Magazine
- South African Medical Journal
- The Lancet
- Rhode Island Medical Journal
- Drug Safety

1.4.3   Conference Proceedings

The conference proceedings that contain articles on human errors in medicine are as follows:

- Proceedings of the Second Annenberg Conference on Enhancing Patient Safety and Reducing Errors in Health Care, 1998.
- Proceedings of the 59th Annual Meeting of the American Society for Information Science, 1996.
- Proceedings of the Annual Human Factors Society Conference, 1998.
- Proceedings of the 17th International Conference of the Systems Safety Society, 1999.
- Proceedings of the First Workshop on Human Error and Clinical Systems (HECS'99), 1999.
- Proceedings of the First Symposium on Human Factors in Medical Devices, 1989.
- Proceedings of the AMIA Annual Fall Symposium, 1986.
- Proceedings of the 6th ISSAT International Conference on Reliability and Quality in Design, 2000.

1.4.4   Organizations

Some of the organizations which provide information on human error in health care are as follows:

- Institute of Medicine, 2001 Wisconsin Avenue NW, Washington, DC 20418, USA.
- American Medical Association, 515 N, State Street, Chicago, Illinois 60610, USA.

- Emergency Care Research Institute (ECRI), 5200 Butler Parkway, Plymouth Meeting, Pennsylvania 19462, USA.
- American Hospital Association (AHA), 840 N, Lake Shore Drive, Chicago, Illinois 60611, USA.
- Food and Drug Administration (FDA), Center for Devices and Radiological Health, 1390 Piccard Drive, Rockville, Maryland 20850, USA.
- Canadian Medical Association, 1867 Alta Vista Drive, Ottawa, Ontario K1G 5W8, Canada.

1.5   Scope of the Book

Just like any other fields, health care is also subjected to human errors. In fact, each year in the United States, the death toll from human error in health care is higher than the combined death toll from breast cancer (42300) and motor vehicle accidents (43500).

More specifically, human error in health care is the eighth leading cause of deaths in the United States. A report entitled "To Err is Human" prepared by the Institute of Medicine (USA) in 1999 calls for greater attention on human errors in the medical field.

Over the years a large number of publications on human error in medicine have surfaced. Almost all of these publications are either journal or conference proceedings articles. There is no book that provides an up-to-date coverage of the subject. This book not only attempts to provide an up-to-date coverage of the on-going efforts on human error in medicine, but it also covers useful developments in the general areas of human reliability and human error. More specifically, the book covers the basics of human factors, human reliability, and human errors in addition to the useful techniques and models in these three areas. Moreover, a chapter on basic mathematical concepts was written to enable readers to better understand its contents as well as the calculations involved.

Finally, the basic objective of this book is to provide information related to human reliability and error to both health care and non-health care professionals. Such information can be useful in minimizing the occurrence of human error in health care. This book will serve as a guide to health care professionals, administrators, students, human factors specialists, biomedical and reliability engineers, as well as safety professionals.

Problems

1. Write an essay on human error in health care.
2. List any five important facts and figures related to human error in the medical field.
3. What is the most important factor, in your opinion, for the increasing attention on human error in health care?
4. What is the difference between human error and an adverse event?
5. Define the following terms:

   - Human reliability
   - Human error
   - Continuous task

6. What is the difference between risk and accident?
7. List at least five important journals for obtaining related information on human error in health care.
8. Define the following terms:

   - Human factors
   - Failure
   - Consequence

References

1. James, B.C. and Hammond, M.E.H., "The Challenge of Variation in Medical Practice," *Archives of Pathology and Laboratory Medicine*, Vol. 124, 2000, pp. 1001–1003.
2. Murry, K., "Canada's Medical Device Industry Faces Cost Pressures, Regulatory Reform," *Med. Dev. Diag. Ind. Mag.*, Vol. 19, No. 8, 1997, pp. 30–39.
3. Perrow, C., *Normal Accidents*, Basic Books, New York, 1984.
4. Beecher, H.K., "The First Anesthesia Death and Some Remarks Suggested by It on the Fields of the Laboratory and the Clinic in the Appraisal of New Anesthetic Agents," *Anesthesiology*, Vol. 2, 1941, pp. 443–449.
5. Cooper, J.B., Newbower, R.S., and Kitz, R.J., "An Analysis of Major Errors and Equipment Failures in Anesthesia Management: Considerations for Prevention and Detection," *Anesthesiology*, Vol. 60, 1984, pp. 34–42.
6. Edwards, G., Morlon, H.J.V., and Pask, E.A., "Deaths Associated with Anesthesia: A Report on 1000 cases," *Anesthesia*, Vol. 11, 1956, pp. 194–220.
7. Cliffton, B.S. and Hotten, W.I.T., "Deaths Associated with Anesthesia," *British Journal of Anesthesia*, Vol. 35, 1963, pp. 250–259.

8. Kohn, L.T., Corrigan, J.M., and Donaldson, M.S. (eds), "To Err Is Human: Building a Safer Health System," *Institute of Medicine Report*, National Academy Press, Washington, D.C., 1999.

9. Dhillon, B.S., "Reliability Technology in Health Care Systems," *Proceedings of the IASTED International Symposium on Computer Advanced Technology in Medicine, Health Care, and Bioengineering*, 1990, pp. 84–87.

10. Chopra, V., Bovill, J.G., Spierdijk, J., and Koornneef, F., "Reported Significant Observations During Anesthesia: Perspective Analysis Over an 18 Month Period," *Br. J. Anaes.*, Vol. 68, 1992, pp. 13–17.

11. Cook, R.I. and Woods, D.D., *Operating at the Sharp End: The Complexity of Human Error, in Human Error in Medicine*, edited by M.S., Bogner, Lawrence Erlbaum Associates Publishers, Hillsdale, New Jersey, 1994, pp. 225–309.

12. Bogner, M.S., *Medical Devices: A New Frontier for Human Factors, CSERIAC Gateway*, Vol. 4, No. 1, 1993, pp. 12–14.

13. Phillips, D.P., Christenfeld, N., and Glynn, L.M., "Increase in U.S. Medication-Error Deaths Between 1983 and 1993," *Lancet*, Vol. 351, 1998, pp. 643–644.

14. Wechsler, J., "Manufacturers Challenged to Reduce Medication Errors," *Pharmaceutical Technology*, February 2000, pp. 14–22.

15. Espinosa, J.A. and Nolan, T.W., "Reducing Errors Made by Emergency Physicians in Interpreting Radiographs: Longitudinal Study," *British Medical Journal*, Vol. 320, 2000, pp. 737–740.

16. Wears, R.L. and Leape, L.L., "Human Error in Emergency Medicine," *Annuals of Emergency Medicine*, Vol. 34, No. 3, 1999, pp. 330–332.

17. Gaba, D.M., "Human Error in Anesthetic Mishaps," *International Anesthesiology Clinics*, Vol. 27, No. 3, 1989, pp. 137–147.

18. Cooper, J.B., "Toward Prevention of Anesthetic Mishaps," *International Anesthesiology Clinics*, Vol. 22, 1984, pp. 167–183.

19. Wright, D., "Critical Incident Reporting in an Intensive Care Unit," *Report*, Western General Hospital, Edinburgh, Scotland, UK, 1999.

20. Roughead, E.E., *et al.*, "Drug-Related Hospital Admissions: A Review of Australian Studies Published 1988–1996," *Med. J. Aust.*, Vol. 168, 1998, pp. 405–408.

21. Smith, D.L., "Medication Errors and DTC Ads.," *Pharmaceutical Executive*, February 2000, pp. 129–130.

22. Bindler, R. and Bayne, T., "Medication Calculation Ability of Registered Nurses," *IMAGE*, Vol. 23, No. 4, 1991, pp. 221–224.

23. Short, T.G., O'Regan, A., Lew, J., and Oh, T.E., "Critical Incident Reporting in an Anesthetic Department Quality Assurance Programme," *Anesthesia*, Vol. 47, 1992, pp. 3–7.

24. Leape, L.L., *The Preventability of Medical Injury, in Human Error in Medicine*, edited by M.S. Bogner, Lawrence Erlbaum Associates, Publishers, Hillsdale, New Jersey, 1994, pp. 13–25.

25. Couch, N.P., *et al.*, "The High Cost of Low-Frequency Events," *New England Journal of Medicine*, Vol. 304, 1981, pp. 634–637.

26. Cooper, J.B., *et al.*, "Preventable Anesthesia Mishaps," *Anesthesiology*, Vol. 49, 1978, pp. 399–406.
27. Davies, J.M. and Strunin, L., "Anesthesia in 1984: How Safe Is It?," *Canadian Medical Association Journal*, Vol. 131, September 1984, pp. 437–441.
28. Omdahl, T.P. (ed), *Reliability, Availability, and Maintainability (RAM) Dictionary*, ASQC, Quality Press, Milwaukee, 1988.
29. Fries, R.C., *Medical Device Quality Assurance and Regulatory Compliance*, Marcel Dekker, Inc., New York, 1998.
30. Gaba, D.M., "Human Error in Dynamic Medical Domains," in *Human Error in Medicine*, edited by M.S. Bogner, Lawrence Erlbaum Associates, Publishers, Hillsdale, New Jersey, 1994, pp. 197–223.
31. Dhillon, B.S., *Human Reliability: with Human Factors*, Pergamon Press, Inc., New York, 1986.
32. Coleman, J.C. and Pharm, D., "Medication Errors: Picking up the Pieces," *Drug Topics*, March 1999, pp. 83–92.

Chapter 2

Human Reliability and Error Mathematics

2.1 Introduction

Mathematics plays an instrumental role in solving various types of science and engineering related problems. Its application ranges from solving interplanetary problems to designing equipment for use in health care. Over the past decades some of the mathematical concepts, in particular probability distributions and stochastic processes (Markov modeling), have been used to study various types of problems in the subject of human reliability and error.

For example, in the late 1960s and early 1970s probability distributions were used to represent the number of times human error occurs, thus predicting the human reliability in performing time-continuous tasks.[1–3] Similarly, the Markov method was used to conduct human performance reliability analysis and to predict the mean time to failure of redundant systems with human errors.[4–6]

This chapter presents various mathematical concepts useful for performing human reliability and error analyses in the health care system.

2.2 Sets and Boolean Algebra Laws

The axiomatic probability is based on set theory and in turn sets are generally called events. Normally, the capital letters are used to represent sets. Two basic set operations are presented below.[7–9]

11

- **Union of sets.** This is denoted by the symbol + or ∪. The union of two sets/events, say X and Y, is the set or event, say Z, that consists of all outcomes that are contained in either of the two events/sets (i.e. X and Y). This is expressed by the following expression:

$$Z = X + Y. \tag{2.1}$$

- **Intersection of sets.** This is denoted by ∩ or a dot (•) or no dot at all. The intersection of two sets/events, say A and B, is the set or event, say C, that consists of all outcomes that are contained in both the events/sets. This is expressed by the following expression:

$$C = A \cap B. \tag{2.2}$$

If there are no common elements between A and B (i.e. $A \cap B = 0$) then sets A and B are known as mutually exclusive or disjoint sets.

Boolean algebra is named after a mathematician named George Boole (1813–1864) and some of its laws are as follows[7]:

$$AA = A, \tag{2.3}$$
$$A + A = A, \tag{2.4}$$
$$A + (AB) = A, \tag{2.5}$$
$$A(AB) = AB, \tag{2.6}$$
$$A(B + C) = (AB) + (AC), \tag{2.7}$$
$$(A + B)(A + C) = A + (BC). \tag{2.8}$$

2.3   Probability Definition and Properties

Probability is defined as[10]:

$$P(A) = \lim_{m \to \infty} \left(\frac{M}{m} \right), \tag{2.9}$$

where

$P(A)$ is the probability of occurrence of event A, and

M is the number of times event A occurs in m repeated experiments.

The basic properties of probability are as follows[7–10]:

- For each event Y, the occurrence probability is:

$$0 \leq P(Y) \leq 1. \tag{2.10}$$

- Probabilities of the sample space S and the negation of the sample space (i.e. $\bar{S}$) are:

$$P(S) = 1, \tag{2.11}$$

and

$$P(\bar{S}) = 0. \tag{2.12}$$

- The probability of an intersection of m independent events is:

$$P(Y_1 Y_2 \cdots Y_m) = P(Y_1)P(Y_2) \cdots P(Y_m), \tag{2.13}$$

where

Y_i is the ith event; for $i = 1, 2, \ldots, m$, and

$P(Y_i)$ is the probability of occurrence of event Y_i; for $i = 1, 2, \ldots, m$.

- The probability of the union of m independent events is:

$$P(Y_1 + Y_2 + \cdots + Y_m) = 1 - \prod_{i=1}^{m}(1 - P(Y_i)). \tag{2.14}$$

For mutually exclusive events, the probability of the union of m events is:

$$P(Y_1 + Y_2 + \cdots + Y_m) = \sum_{i=1}^{m} P(Y_i). \tag{2.15}$$

- The probability of occurrence and nonoccurrence of an event, say Y, is:

$$P(Y) + P(\bar{Y}) = 1, \tag{2.16}$$

where

$P(Y)$ is the probability of occurrence of Y, and

$P(\bar{Y})$ is the probability of nonoccurrence of Y.

Example 2.1   Assume that a medical task is performed by two independent individuals. The task will be performed incorrectly if either of the individuals makes an error. The probability of making an error by the individual is 0.2. Calculate the probability that the task will not be accomplished successfully.

Substituting the given data values into Eq. 2.14 yields:

$$P(Y_1 + Y_2) = 1 - \prod_{i=1}^{2}(1 - P(Y_i))$$
$$= P(Y_i) + P(Y_2) - P(Y_1)P(Y_2)$$
$$= 0.2 + 0.2 - (0.2)(0.2)$$
$$= 0.36.$$

There is a 36% chance that the task will not be accomplished successfully.

Example 2.2   In Example 2.1, calculate the probability that the task will be performed successfully.   Also, prove that the total probability of accomplishing and not accomplishing the task successfully is equal to unity.

Using Eq. 2.16, the probability of not making an error by the individual is

$$R = 1 - 0.2$$
$$= 0.8,$$

where R is the individual's reliability.

The task will only be accomplished successfully, if both the individuals do not commit any error. Thus, using the above-calculated value and the specified data in Eq. 2.13 we get:

$$P(Y_1Y_2) = P(Y_1)P(Y_2)$$
$$= (0.8)(0.8)$$
$$= 0.64.$$

Thus, the probability that the task will be accomplished successfully is 0.64. By adding this value to the one calculated in Example 2.1 proves that the total probability of accomplishing and not accomplishing the task successfully is equal to unity.

2.4   Discrete Random Variables and Probability Distributions

If X is a random variable on the sample space S along with a countable infinite set $X(S) = \{x_1, x_2, x_3, x_4, \ldots\}$, then all these random variables along with the other finite sets are known as discrete random variables.[11]

For a single-dimension discrete random variable, say X, the discrete probability density function of that random variable is denoted by $f(x_i)$ if the following conditions apply:

$$f(x_i) \geq 0, \text{ for all } x_i \in R_x \text{(range space), and} \tag{2.17}$$

$$\sum f(x_i) = 1, \text{ for all } x_i. \tag{2.18}$$

Similarly, the cumulative probability or distribution function is defined by

$$F(x) = \sum_{x_i \leq x} f(x_i), \tag{2.19}$$

where $F(x)$ is the cumulative distribution function.

The value of $F(x)$ is always

$$0 \leq F(x) \leq 1. \tag{2.20}$$

Some of the discrete random variable probability distributions are presented below.

2.4.1   *Binomial Distribution*

This distribution is also known as the Bernoulli distribution, named after its originator, Jakob Bernoulli (1654–1705). The distribution is used in situations when one is concerned with the probabilities of outcome such as the total number of failures (errors) in a sequence of m trials.

The distribution is based on the condition that each trial has two possible outcomes, success and failure, and the probability of each trial remains constant. The distribution probability density function is defined by:

$$f(y) = \frac{m}{y!(m-y)!} p^y q^{m-y}, \quad y = 0, 1, 2, \ldots, m, \tag{2.21}$$

where

y is the total number of failures (errors) in m trials,

q is the probability of failure of a single trial, and

p is the probability of success of a single trial.

The cumulative distribution function is given by:

$$F(y) = \sum_{i=0}^{y} \binom{m}{i} p^i q^{m-i}, \qquad (2.22)$$

where

$$\binom{m}{i} = \frac{m!}{i!(m-i)!}, \text{ and}$$

$F(y)$ is the probability of y or less failures (errors) in m total trials.

The mean and variance of the distribution, respectively, are as follows[12]:

$$\mu_b = mp, \text{ and} \qquad (2.23)$$
$$\sigma_b^2 = mpq, \qquad (2.24)$$

where

μ_b is the mean of the binomial distribution, and

σ_b^2 is the variance of the binomial distribution.

2.4.2   *Poisson Distribution*

This distribution is named after Simeon Poisson (1781–1840).[13] The distribution is applied in situations when one is concerned with the occurrence of a number of events that are of the same kind. The occurrence of an event is represented as a point on a time scale and in reliability work each event denotes a failure (error). The distribution density function is defined by:

$$f(m) = \frac{(\theta t)^m e^{-\theta t}}{m!}, \quad m = 0, 1, 2, \ldots, \qquad (2.25)$$

where

θ is the constant arrival, failure, or error rate, and

t is time.

The cumulative distribution function is given by:

$$F = \sum_{i=0}^{m} \frac{(\theta t)^i e^{-\theta t}}{i!}.$$

(2.26)

The mean and variance of the Poisson distribution, respectively, are as follows[8]:

$$\mu_p = \theta t, \text{ and}$$

(2.27)

$$\sigma_p^2 = \theta t,$$

(2.28)

where

μ_p is the mean of the Poisson distribution, and

σ_p^2 is the variance of the Poisson distribution.

2.4.3   *Geometric Distribution*

This distribution is based on the same assumptions as the binomial distribution, except that the number of trials is not fixed. More specifically, the trials are conducted until a success is achieved.[9,14] Again, with respect to the assumptions, all trials are identical and independent, and each can result in one of the two possible outcomes (i.e. a success or a failure (error)).

The geometric probability density function is defined by:

$$f(y) = pq^{y-1}, \quad y = 0, 1, 2, 3, \ldots.$$

(2.29)

The cumulative distribution function is given by[9]:

$$F(y) = \begin{cases} 0, & y < 1. \\ \sum pq^{y_i - 1}, & y \geq 1. \\ y_i \leq [y]. \end{cases}$$

(2.30)

The mean and variance of the geometric distribution, respectively, are:

$$\mu_g = \frac{1}{p}, \text{ and}$$

(2.31)

$$\sigma_g^2 = \frac{q}{p^2},$$

(2.32)

where

μ_g is the mean of the geometric distribution, and

σ_g^2 is the variance of the geometric distribution.

2.5   Continuous Random Variables and Probability Distributions

A real-valued function defined over a sample space S is known as a continuous random variable. Probability density and cumulative distribution functions of the continuous random variable are defined respectively as follows[10,11]:

$$f(t) = \frac{dF(t)}{dt}, \text{ and} \tag{2.33}$$

$$F(t) = \int_{-\infty}^{t} f(x)\,dx, \tag{2.34}$$

where

$f(t)$ is the probability density function of the continuous random variable t.

$F(t)$ is the cumulative distribution function of the continuous random variable t.

As t becomes very large, from Eq. 2.34 we get

$$F(\infty) = 1. \tag{2.35}$$

The expected value, $E(t)$, of a continuous random variable is defined by:

$$E(t) = \int_{-\infty}^{\infty} tf(t)\,dt. \tag{2.36}$$

In reliability work when t represents time the expected value is known as the mean time to failure (MTTF) or the mean time to human error (MTTHE). Thus, from Eq. 2.26, we get:

$$\text{MTTHE} = \int_{0}^{\infty} tf(t)\,dt. \tag{2.37}$$

Using Eq. 2.37, we obtain the following alternative formula for MTTHE[15]:

$$\text{MTTHE} = \int_{0}^{\infty} R(t)\,dt, \tag{2.38}$$

where

$R(t)$ is the reliability function and is defined by:

$$R(t) = 1 - F(t)$$

$$= 1 - \int_{-\infty}^{t} f(x)\, dx. \tag{2.39}$$

Occasionally in reliability work Eq. 2.29 is simply written as:

$$R(t) = 1 - \int_{0}^{t} f(x)\, dx, \quad \text{or} \tag{2.40}$$

$$R(t) = \int_{t}^{\infty} f(x)\, dx. \tag{2.41}$$

The continuous random variable probability distributions considered useful for performing human reliability and error analyses in health care are presented in the following subsections.[8–12]

2.5.1 *Exponential Distribution*

This is the most widely used distribution in reliability work and is one of the simplest distributions used in performing practically inclined reliability analyses.

The distribution probability density function is defined by:

$$f(t) = \lambda e^{-\lambda t} \quad t \geq 0, \ \lambda > 0, \tag{2.42}$$

where

t is time,

λ is the distribution parameter. In human reliability work, it is known as the error rate, and

$f(t)$ is the probability density function.

By substituting Eq. 2.42 into Eq. 2.34 the following expression for the cumulative distribution function is obtained:

$$F(t) = \int_{-\infty}^{t} \lambda e^{-\lambda x}\, dx$$

$$= 1 - e^{-\lambda t}. \tag{2.43}$$

Substituting Eq. 2.42 into Eq. 2.40, we get the following expression for the reliability function:

$$R(t) = 1 - \int_0^t \lambda e^{-\lambda x} \, dx$$

$$= e^{-\lambda t}. \tag{2.44}$$

With the aid of Eqs. 2.36 and 2.42, the following expression for the expected or mean value of t was obtained:

$$E(t) = \frac{1}{\lambda}. \tag{2.45}$$

When the value of λ is in terms of human errors/unit time (e.g. errors/hour), Eq. 2.45 gives the MTTHE.

Example 2.3   A medical professional is performing a certain task and his/her error rate is 0.004 errors/hour. Calculate the professional's reliability for a 7-hour mission and the mean time to human error.

Substituting the given data into Eq. 2.44 yields:

$$R(7) = e^{-(0.004)(7)}$$

$$= 0.9724.$$

Similarly, using the given error rate value in Eq. 2.45, we get:

$$E(t) = \text{MTTHE} = \frac{1}{0.004}$$

$$= 250 \text{ hours}.$$

Thus, the professional's reliability and MTTHE are 0.9724 and 250 hours, respectively.

2.5.2   Rayleigh Distribution

This distribution is used in reliability analysis when an item's failure rate or a person's error rate increases linearly with time. The distribution probability density function is defined by:

$$f(t) = \frac{2}{\alpha^2} t e^{-(t/\alpha)^2} \quad t \geq 0, \ \alpha > 0, \tag{2.46}$$

where α is the distribution parameter.

Substituting Eq. 2.46 into Eq. 2.34 yields the following expression for the cumulative distribution function:

$$F(t) = \int_{-\infty}^{t} \frac{2}{\alpha^2} x e^{-(x/\alpha)^2} dx$$

$$= 1 - e^{-(t/\alpha)^2}. \tag{2.47}$$

By inserting Eq. 2.46 into Eq. 2.36, we obtain the following expression for the expected or the mean value of t:

$$E(t) = \alpha \Gamma \left(\frac{3}{2} \right), \tag{2.48}$$

where $\Gamma(\bullet)$ is the gamma function and is defined by:

$$\Gamma(y) = \int_{0}^{\infty} t^{y-1} e^{-t} dt, \quad \text{for } y > 0. \tag{2.49}$$

2.5.3   *Weibull Distribution*

This distribution was developed by W. Weibull, a Swedish mechanical engineering professor, in the early 1950s.[16] It is a widely used distribution to represent many different physical phenomena. The probability density function for the distribution is expressed by:

$$f(t) = \frac{\beta t^{\beta-1}}{\alpha^\beta} e^{-(t/\alpha)^\beta}, \quad t \geq 0, \ \beta > 0, \ \alpha > 0, \tag{2.50}$$

where α and β are the distribution scale and shape parameters, respectively.

By substituting Eq. 2.50 into Eq. 2.34, we get the following expression for the cumulative distribution function:

$$F(t) = \int_{-\infty}^{t} \frac{\beta x^{\beta-1}}{\alpha^\beta} e^{-(x/\alpha)^\beta} dx$$

$$= 1 - e^{-(t/\alpha)^\beta}. \tag{2.51}$$

Substituting Eq. 2.50 into Eq. 2.36 yields the following expression for the expected or mean value of t:

$$E(t) = \alpha \Gamma \left(1 + \frac{1}{\beta} \right). \tag{2.52}$$

when for $\beta = 1$ and 2, Eqs. 2.50–2.52 become equations for the exponential and the Rayleigh distributions, respectively. Thus, the exponential and the Rayleigh distributions are special cases of the Weibull distribution.

2.5.4   *Normal Distribution*

This is a widely used distribution and occasionally it is also referred to as the Gaussian distribution after Carl F. Gauss (1777–1855), a German mathematician. The distribution probability density function is defined by:

$$f(t) = \frac{1}{\sigma\sqrt{2\pi}} \exp\left[-\frac{(t-\mu)^2}{2\sigma^2}\right], \quad -\infty < t < +\infty, \qquad (2.53)$$

where

μ is the distribution parameter known as the mean value.

σ is the distribution parameter known as the standard deviation.

Substituting Eq. 2.53 into Eq. 2.34 yields the following expression for the cumulative distribution function:

$$F(t) = \frac{1}{\sigma\sqrt{2\pi}} \int_{-\infty}^{t} \exp\left[-\frac{(x-\mu)}{2\sigma^2}\right] dx. \qquad (2.54)$$

By substituting Eq. 2.53 into Eq. 2.36, we get the following expression for the expected value of t:

$$E(t) = \mu. \qquad (2.55)$$

2.5.5   *Gamma Distribution*

This is a two-parameter distribution and is quite flexible in fitting a wide variety of problems including human reliability and error. The probability density function of the distribution is defined by:

$$f(t) = \frac{\lambda(\lambda t)^{\theta-1}}{\Gamma(\theta)} e^{-\lambda t}, \quad t \geq 0, \ \lambda, \ \theta > 0, \qquad (2.56)$$

where

λ and θ are the distribution scale and the shape parameters, respectively, and

$\Gamma(\bullet)$ is the gamma function.

By substituting Eq. 2.56 into Eq. 2.34, we get the following expression for the cumulative distribution function[11,15]:

$$F(t) = \int_{-\infty}^{t} \frac{\lambda(\lambda x)^{\theta-1}}{\Gamma(\theta)} e^{-\lambda x} \, dx$$

$$= 1 - \sum_{i=0}^{\theta-1} \frac{e^{-\lambda t}(\lambda t)^i}{i!}. \tag{2.57}$$

Substituting Eq. 2.56 into Eq. 2.36 yields the following expression for the expected value of t:

$$E(t) = \frac{\theta}{\lambda}. \tag{2.58}$$

For $\theta = 1$, the gamma distribution becomes the exponential distribution.

2.6 Laplace Transform Definition and Final Value Theorem

The Laplace transform of the function $f(t)$ is defined by:

$$F(s) = \int_{0}^{\infty} f(t) e^{-st} \, dt, \tag{2.59}$$

where

t is the time random variable,

s is the Laplace transform variable, and

$F(s)$ is the Laplace transform of $f(t)$.

Example 2.4   Obtain the Laplace transform of the following function:

$$f(t) = e^{-bt}, \tag{2.60}$$

where b is a constant.

Substituting Eq. 2.60 into Eq. 2.59 yields:

$$F(s) = \int_{0}^{\infty} e^{-bt} e^{-st} \, dt$$

$$= -\frac{e^{-(s+b)t}}{(s+b)} \Big|_{0}^{\infty}$$

$$= \frac{1}{s+b}. \tag{2.61}$$

Table 2.1.   Laplace transforms of selected functions.

No.	$f(t)$	$F(s)$
1	K (a constant)	K/s
2	$e^{-\lambda t}$	$1/(s + \lambda)$
3	t^m, for $m = 0, 1, 2, \ldots$	$m!/s^{m+1}$
4	$\dfrac{df(t)}{dt}$	$sF(s) - f(0)$

Table 2.1 presents the Laplace transforms of selective functions considered useful for performing human reliability analyses.[17]

The Laplace transform of the final value theorem is expressed as follows[15]:

$$\lim_{t \to \infty} f(t) = \lim_{s \to 0} [sF(s)]. \tag{2.62}$$

Example 2.5   Obtain the steady state value of the following function:

$$f(t) = \frac{\mu}{\lambda + \mu} + \frac{\lambda}{\lambda + \mu} e^{-(\lambda + \mu)t}, \tag{2.63}$$

where λ and μ are the constants.

By substituting Eq. 2.63 into Eq. 2.59, the following equation is obtained:

$$F(s) = \frac{\mu}{(\lambda + \mu)s} + \frac{\lambda}{(\lambda + \mu)} \cdot \frac{1}{(s + \lambda + \mu)}. \tag{2.64}$$

Substituting Eq. 2.64 into the right hand side of Eq. 2.62 yields:

$$f_{ss} = \frac{\mu}{\lambda + \mu}, \tag{2.65}$$

where f_{ss} is the steady value of Eq. 2.63.

2.7   Differential Equation Solution

Many a time in order to perform human reliability/error analyses, the solutions to a set of differential equations will have to be found. The use of Laplace transforms is considered an effective approach for finding the solutions to the type of differential equations occurring in human reliability work. The following example demonstrates the application of Laplace transforms in finding the solutions to a first order differential equation:

Example 2.6 Find the solution to the following differential equation using Laplace transforms:

$$\frac{df(t)}{dt} + \lambda f(t) = 0, \qquad (2.66)$$

where λ is a constant.

At time $t = 0$, $f(0) = 1$.

Using the Laplace transforms, we write Eq. 2.66 in the following form:

$$sF(s) - f(0) + \lambda F(s) = 0. \qquad (2.67)$$

Using the initial conditions and rearranging Eq. 2.67 yields:

$$F(s) = \frac{1}{s + \lambda}. \qquad (2.68)$$

Taking the inverse Laplace transform of Eq. 2.68 yields the following expression:

$$f(t) = e^{-\lambda t}. \qquad (2.69)$$

Thus, Eq. 2.69 is the solution to Eq. 2.66.

Problems

1. Prove the following law of Boolean algebra:

$$(A + B)(A + C) = A + BC. \qquad (2.70)$$

2. Write down four basic properties of probability.
3. Make a comparison between independent and mutually exclusive events.
4. Assume that a medical task is performed by two independent individuals. The task will be performed incorrectly if either of the individuals makes an error. The probability of making an error by the individual is 0.1. Calculate the probability that the task will not be accomplished successfully.
5. What is the difference between discrete and continuous random variables?

6. Write down the probability density functions of two discrete random variable distributions.
7. Prove that the total area under a probability density function curve is equal to unity.
8. Define cumulative distribution function.
9. Prove that Eqs. 2.37 and 2.38 give the same results.
10. Obtain the Laplace transform of the following function:

$$f(t) = t^{\alpha}, \quad \text{for } \alpha = 0, 1, 2, 3, \ldots, \qquad (2.71)$$

where t is a variable.

References

1. Askren, W.B. and Regulinski, T.L., "Quantifying Human Performance for Reliability Analysis of Systems," *Human Factors*, Vol. 11, 1969, pp. 393–396.
2. Regulinski, T.L. and Askren, W.B., "Mathematical Modeling of Human Performance Reliability," *Proceedings of the Annual Symposium on Reliability*, 1969, pp. 5–11.
3. Regulinski, T.L. and Askren, W.B., "Stochastic Modeling of Human Performance Effectiveness Functions," *Proceedings of the Annual Reliability and Maintainability Symposium*, 1972, pp. 407–416.
4. Dhillon, B.S., "System Reliability Evaluation Models with Human Errors," *IEEE Transactions on Reliability*, Vol. 32, 1983, pp. 47–48.
5. Dhillon, B.S., "Stochastic Models for Predicting Human Reliability," *Microelectronics and Reliability*, Vol. 25, 1982, pp. 491–496.
6. Dhillon, B.S. and Rayapati, S.N., "Reliability Analysis of Non-Maintained Parallel Systems Subject to Hardware Failure and Human Error," *Microelectronics and Reliability*, Vol. 25, 1985, pp. 111–122.
7. Lipschutz, S., *Set Theory and Related Topics*, McGraw-Hill Book Company, New York, 1964.
8. Shooman, M.L., *Probabilistic Reliability*, McGraw-Hill Book Company, New York, 1968.
9. Montgomery, D.C. and Runger, G.C., *Applied Statistics and Probability for Engineers*, John Wiley and Sons, Inc., New York, 1999.
10. Mann, N.R., Schafer, R.E., and Singpurwalla, N.D., *Methods for Statistical Analysis of Reliability and Life Data*, John Wiley and Sons, New York, 1974.
11. Dhillon, B.S. and Singh, C., *Engineering Reliability: New Techniques and Applications*, John Wiley and Sons, New York, 1981.
12. Patel, J.K., Kapadia, C.H., and Owen, D.B., *Handbook of Statistical Distributions*, Marcel Dekker, Inc., New York, 1976.
13. Eves, H., *An Introduction to the History of Mathematics*, Holt, Rinehart and Winston, Inc., New York, 1976.

14. Tsokos, C.P., *Probability Distributions: An Introduction to Probability Theory with Applications*, Wadsworth Publishing Company, Belmont, California, 1972.
15. Dhillon, B.S., *Mechanical Reliability: Theory, Models, and Applications*, American Institute of Aeronautics and Astronautics, Washington, D.C., 1988.
16. Weibull, W., "A Statistical Distribution Function of Wide Applicability," *Journal of Applied Mechanics*, Vol. 18, 1951, pp. 293–297.
17. Oberhettinger, F. and Badii, L., *Tables of Laplace Transforms*, Springer-Verlag, New York, 1973.

Chapter 3

Human Factors Basics

3.1 Introduction

The history of human factors dates back to 1898, when Frederick W. Taylor performed various studies to determine the most suitable design of shovels.[1] In 1911, Frank B. Gilbreth studied the problem of bricklaying and invented the scaffold.[2,3] The use of scaffold almost tripled the number of bricks laid per hour (i.e. from 120 to 350 bricks per hour). In 1918, the United States Department of Defense established laboratories for conducting researches on various human factors-related areas at the Brooks and Wright–Patterson Air Force Bases.[4]

In 1924, the National Research Council (USA) initiated a study concerned with the various aspects of human relations (e.g. investigating the effects of varying illumination, length of workday, and rest periods on productivity) at the Hawthorne Plant of Western Electric in the State of Illinois. By the end of World War II, human factors or human factors engineering came to be recognized as a specialized discipline. In 1954, a database on body dimensions using United States Air Force (USAF) personnel as subjects, was developed by Hertzberg *et al.*[5] In 1972, the United States Department of Defense released a military document on human factors.[6]

Over the years, a vast number of publications on human factors have surfaced and today, it is a well developed field in the world. This chapter presents the important fundamental aspects of human factors.

3.2   Man-Machine System Types and Comparisons

Although, there are many different types of man-machine systems, they can be grouped under three categories as shown in Fig. 3.1.[7]

The manual systems are composed of hand tools and other aids along with the human operator who controls the operation. This operator uses his/her own physical energy as a power source, and then he/she transmits or receives from these tools a great amount of information. The automated systems perform all operation-related functions including decision making, sensing, action, and processing. Most of these systems are of the closed-loop type (a closed-loop system may be described as a continuous system performing some processes that require continuous control and appropriate feedback for its successful operational mission). Usually, the basic human functions associated with the automated systems are programming, monitoring, and maintenance.

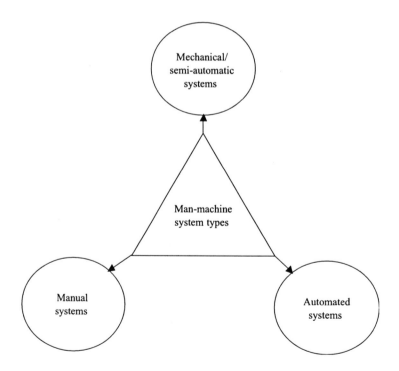

Fig. 3.1.   Types of man-machine systems.

The mechanical or semi automatic systems are composed of well-integrated physical parts, such as various types of powered machine tools. Typically in these systems the machines provide the power and the human operator basically performs the control function.

Many times during the design phase of a system decisions will have to be made on whether to assign certain functions to the machines or to humans. Under such a scenario, an effective knowledge on the capabilities/limitations of humans and machines is very important. Some comparisons of human and machine capabilities/limitations are presented in Table 3.1.[8]

3.3 Human Behaviors

Various studies conducted over the years have confirmed that humans have built-in tendencies towards certain objects and their motor/behavioral development varies with age. In order to minimize the occurrence of human errors, the findings such as these must be carefully considered during the design and development of medical related products.

This section focuses on the typical human behaviors along with the corresponding important design considerations as well as the behaviors toward safety for the different age groups.

3.3.1 *Typical Human Behaviors and the Corresponding Design Considerations*

Some of the expected human behaviors and the corresponding design considerations in the parentheses are:

- Humans get easily confused with unfamiliar things (avoid designing completely unfamiliar items).
- Humans have become accustomed to certain color meanings (strictly observe existing color-coding standards during design).
- Humans' attention is drawn towards items such as loud noise, flashing lights, bright lights, as well as bright and vivid colors (design in stimuli of appropriate intensity when attention requires stimulation).
- Humans expect that valve handles/faucets will rotate counterclockwise to increase the flow of liquid, steam, or gas (design such items according to human expectations).

Table 3.1.   Human and machine capability/limitation comparisons.

No.	Human	Machine
1	Is subjected to social environments of all types.	Is independent of social environments of all kinds.
2	Is very flexible with regards to task performance.	Is relatively quite inflexible.
3	Has an excellent memory.	Is remarkably costly to have the same capability.
4	Is subjected to factors such as disorientation, motion sickness, and coriolis effects.	Is totally free of such effects.
5	Is subjected to stress because of interpersonal or other problems.	Is totally free of such problems.
6	Is limited to a certain degree in channel capacity.	Can have unlimited channel capacities.
7	Has relatively easy maintenance requirements.	Maintenance problems become serious with the increase in complexity.
8	Is subjected to deterioration in performance because of boredom and fatigue.	Is not affected by factors such as these, but its performance is subjected to deterioration because of wear or lack of calibration.
9	Is affected adversely by high g forces.	Is totally independent of g forces.
10	Has rather restricted short-term memory for factual matters.	Can have unlimited short-term memory but its affordability is a limiting factor.
11	Is very capable of making inductive decisions under novel conditions.	Has very little or no induction capabilities at all.
12	Is frequently subjected to departure from following an optimum strategy.	Always follows the design strategy.
13	Has tolerance for factors such as uncertainty, vagueness, and ambiguity.	Is quite limited in tolerance with respect to factors such as these.
14	Is quite unsuitable for carrying out tasks such as transformation, amplification, or data coding.	Is extremely useful for carrying out tasks such as these.
15	Performance efficiency is affected by anxiety.	Is quite independent of this shortcoming.
16	Is a poor monitor of events that do not occur frequently.	Possesses an option to be designed to reliably detect infrequently occurring events.

• Humans will frequently use their sense of touch to explore or test the unknown (pay special attention to this factor during design, particularly to the product handling aspect).

- Humans often regard manufactured items as being safe (place emphasis on designing products so that they become impossible to be used incorrectly).
- Humans expect that to turn on the power, the electrically powered switches have to move upward, or to the right, etc. (design such items according to human expectations).
- Humans often tend to hurry (develop design so that it takes into consideration the element of human hurry).
- Humans usually possess very little knowledge about their physical shortcomings (develop appropriate design by carefully considering human basic characteristics and shortcomings).[9]

3.3.2   *Behavior Towards Safety for the Different Age Groups*

Past experiences show that human behavior towards safety varies with age. Some of the typical human behaviors towards safety for the different age groups in the parentheses are: the tendency to move slowly and cautiously when engaging in all activities, lacking patience, being unaware of obvious hazards, etc. (senior citizens), the tendency to take relatively less risks and to exercise greater caution (older adults and persons close to their retirement age), the tendency to take only well-calculated risks and orientation towards efficiency and cost (early and middle years of adulthood), the tendency to use newly acquired strength, take chances, etc. (young adults), the tendency towards erratic behavior, resistance to authority, etc. (teenage children), the tendency to take chances in order to be accepted by the peer group (school-age children), and the tendency to be curious about anything and everything (infants and young children).[9]

3.4   Human Sensory Capacities

As humans possess many useful sensors (i.e. sight, touch, smell, taste, and hearing), a better understanding of their sensory capacities can help to reduce the occurrence of errors in health care. This section discusses the effects of sight, noise, touch, and vibration in separate subsections.[10]

3.4.1   *Sight*

This is stimulated by the electromagnetic radiation of specific wavelengths, frequently referred to as the visible portion of the electromagnetic spectrum.

The various areas of the spectrum, as seen by the human eye, appear to vary in brightness. For example, during the day, the human eye is most sensitive to greenish-yellow light with a wavelength of around 5500 Angstrom units.[10] In addition, the eye sees differently from different angles. Furthermore, the eye perceives all colors when it is looking straight ahead but as the viewing angle increases, the color perception starts to decrease.

Some of the additional factors associated with color are as follows[10]:

- Color-weak people do not see colors in a similar manner as normal individuals do.
- In poorly illuminated places or at night, color differences are very minimal. In particular, from a distant or for a small point source (e.g. a small warning light), it is impossible to make a clear distinction between orange, green, blue, and yellow. In fact, they will all appear to be white.
- Staring at a certain colored light and then glancing away may lead to the reversal of color in the brain. For example, to stare at a green or red light and then glance away, the signal to the brain may totally reverse the color.

Three important sight-related guidelines are as follows:

- Do not rely too much on color where critical activities may be performed by fatigued individuals.
- Choose the right color so that color-weak people do not get confused.
- Use red filters, if possible, with wavelengths longer than 6500 Angstrom units.

3.4.2 *Noise*

Noise may be described as sounds that lack coherence and its effects on humans are difficult to be gaged precisely. Past experiences indicate that human reactions to noise extend beyond the auditory systems (i.e. to feelings such as well-being, fatigue, irritability, or boredom). Moreover, excessive noise can result in various types of problems including the loss of hearing if exposed for long periods, the reduction in the workers' efficiency, and the adverse effects on tasks requiring a high degree of muscular coordination and precision or intense concentration.

Usually, two major physical characteristics (i.e. intensity and frequency) are used to describe noise. Intensity is normally measured in decibels (dB) and an individual exposed to over 80 dB of noise can suffer from temporary/permanent loss of hearing. Intensity levels for noise sources such as motion picture sound studio, voice whisper, quiet residential area, household ventilation fan, normal conversation, and heavy traffic are 10 dB, 20 dB, 40 dB, 56 dB, 60 dB, and 70 dB, respectively.[7,11]

In the case of frequency, the human ear is most sensitive to frequencies in the range of 600–900 Hz and it has the capacity to detect sounds of frequencies from 20–20000 Hz. Normally, humans suffer a major loss of hearing when they are exposed to noise frequencies between 4000 and 6000 Hz for long period of time.[10,11]

3.4.3 *Touch*

The sense of touch is closely associated with the ability of humans in interpreting auditory and visual stimuli. The sensory cues received by the skin and muscles can be employed to a certain degree to send messages to the brain, thus relieving the eyes and the ears a part of the work load. In situations when a human user is expected to rely totally on his/her touch sensors, different knob shapes could be adopted for use.

Nonetheless, the use of the touch sensor in various technical-related tasks is not new; in fact it has been employed for centuries by craft workers to detect surface roughness and irregularities in their work. Various studies conducted over the years indicated that the detection accuracy of surface irregularities improves quite dramatically when the individual moves an intermediate thin cloth or a piece of paper over the object surface instead of just using bare fingers.[12]

3.4.4 *Vibration*

The presence of vibration could be detrimental to the performance of both physical and mental tasks by humans. There are various parameters of vibrations including amplitude, frequency, acceleration, and velocity. In particular, large amplitude and low frequency vibrations contribute to problems such as eyestrain, motion sickness, fatigue, headaches, and interference with the ability to read and interpret instruments.[10] These symptoms become less pronounced as the amplitude of vibration decreases and the frequency increases. Nonetheless, low amplitude and high frequency vibrations can also be quite fatiguing. Some important guidelines for lowering the effects of vibration and motion are as follows[10,13]:

- Make use of damping materials or cushioned seats for reducing vibrations transmitted to a seated individual and avoid vibrations of frequencies 3 to 4 Hz as this is the resonant frequency of a vertically seated person.
- Eliminate, if possible, vibrations in excess of 0.08 mil amplitude.
- Resist vibrations and shocks through appropriate designs or isolate them by using items such as shock absorbers, springs, fluid couplings, or cushioned mountings.

3.5   Human Body Measurements

Since most engineering products are operated and maintained by humans, information on their body measurements is crucial to designers for allocating appropriate workspace and tasks to the involved individuals. Usually, the human body related requirements are outlined in the product design specification, particularly if the product is to be used by military personnels. For example, the United States Department of Defense MIL-STD-1472 clearly states that "design shall insure operability and maintainability by at least 90% of the user population and the design range shall include at least the 5th and the 95th percentiles for design-critical body dimensions".[14]

The standard or document also specifies that the use of anthropometries data should take into consideration factors such as the nature and frequency of tasks to be performed, the tasks' flexibility needs, the position of the body during the task performance, the difficulties associated with the intended tasks, and the increments in the design-critical dimensions imposed by protective garments.

The following are the two basic sources for obtaining information on body measurements[10]:

- **Anthropometrics surveys.** In this case measurements of a sample of the population are taken and these data are usually presented in the form of percentiles, ranges, and means.
- **Experiments.** In this case, the conditions in question are simulated by experiments and then the required data are collected.

The body measurements are grouped under two categories: dynamics and static. The dynamic measurements usually vary with body movements and they include those taken with subjects in different working positions, as well as different leg and arm reaches. The static measurements incorporate everything ranging from the measurements of the most gross aspects of the body size to the measurements of the distance between the pupils of the eyes.

Tables 3.2 and 3.3 present the structural body dimensions and the weights of both male and female US adults (18 to 79 years), respectively.[7–9,14]

Table 3.2. Some selected body dimensions and weights of male US adults (18 to 79 years).

No.	Body Feature	Percentile*	
		5th	95th
1	Seat breadth	12.2	15.9
2	Weight	126	217
3	Height, standing	63.8	72.8
4	Height, sitting normal	31.6	36.6
5	Seated eye height	28.7	33.5
6	Knee height	19.3	23.4
7	Elbow-to-elbow breadth	13.7	19.9
8	Height, sitting erect	33.2	38

*Dimensions given in inches and weight in pounds.

Table 3.3. Some selected body dimensions and weights of female US adults (18 to 79 years).

No.	Body Feature	Percentile*	
		5th	95th
1	Seat breadth	12.3	17.1
2	Weight	104	199
3	Height, standing	59	67.1
4	Height, sitting normal	29.6	34.7
5	Seated eye height	27.4	31.0
6	Knee height	17.9	21.5
7	Elbow-to-elbow breadth	12.3	19.3
8	Height, sitting erect	30.9	35.7

*Dimensions given in inches and weight in pounds.

3.6   Human Factors-Related Formulas

After conducting extensive research, human factors specialists have developed various types of mathematical formulas for making a variety of decisions. Many of these formulas can also be used in the health care area. This section presents some of these formulas considered useful for applications in the medical system.

3.6.1   *Character Height Estimation Formula I*

This formula was developed by Peters and Adams in 1959 and is concerned with the estimation of character height by considering various factors including illumination, viewing distance, viewing conditions, and the importance of reading accuracy.[15] Thus, the character height in inches is expressed by:

$$H_C = \theta D + CF_I + CF_{II}, \tag{3.1}$$

where

H_C is the character height in inches,

CF_I is the correction factor for importance. Its recommended value for emergency labels or similar items is 0.075 and for other items $CF_I = 0$,

D is the viewing distance expressed in inches,

θ is a constant with the specified value of 0.0022, and

CF_{II} is the correction factor for viewing and illumination conditions. The recommended values of this factor for different conditions are: 0.06 (above a 1 foot-candle and favorable reading conditions), 0.26 (below a 1 foot-candle and unfavorable reading conditions), 0.16 (above a 1 foot-candle and unfavorable reading conditions), and 0.16 (below a 1 foot-candle and favorable reading conditions).

Example 3.1   The estimated viewing distance of an instrument panel is 50 inches and after a careful consideration, the values of CF_I and CF_{II} were decided to be 0.075 and 0.26, respectively. Compute the height of the label characters to be used at the panel.

By inserting the specified data values into Eq. 3.1, we get

$$H_C = (0.0022)(50) + 0.075 + 0.26$$
$$= 0.445 \text{ inches.}$$

It means that the height of the label characters to be used is 0.445 inches.

3.6.2 *Character Height Estimation Formula II*

Usually the instrument panels are located at a viewing distance of 28 inches for the comfortable performance and control of adjustment-oriented tasks. More specifically, the viewing distance of 28 inches is often used to determine the sizes of letters, markings, and numbers. For a viewing distance other than 28 inches, the following formula can be used to estimate character height[7,16]:

$$NC_h = \frac{(SCH)(RVD)}{28}, \tag{3.2}$$

where

    RVD   is the required viewing distance in inches,

    SCH   is the standard character height from a viewing distance of 28 inches, and

    NC_h is the new height of a character at RVD specified in inches.

Example 3.2   A meter at an instrument panel has to be read from a distance of 56 inches and the standard character height at a viewing distance of 28 inches is 0.30 inches. Calculate the height of the numerals for the specified viewing distance.

Substituting the given values into Eq. 3.2 yields:

$$NC_h = \frac{(0.30)(56)}{28}$$
$$= 0.6 \text{ inches.}$$

Thus, the height of numerals for the specified viewing distance of 56 inches is 0.6 inches.

3.6.3 *Noise Reduction Estimation Formula*

Noise could be a major problem in various facilities including health care; thus its reduction is absolutely essential. Factors such as transmission loss, absorption properties of walls in the receiving room, and the area of the walls capable of transmitting sound play an important role in noise reduction. Thus, the total noise reduction can be estimated by using the following formula[16]:

$$NR = \alpha + \log(P_a/A_w), \tag{3.3}$$

where

NR   is the total noise reduction,

A_w is the total area of wall transmitting sound in ft^2,

P_a is the total absorption properties of walls in the noise receiving room, and

α is the transmission loss of materials of varying thickness in decibels. Nonetheless, α is defined by the following equation:

$$\alpha = \frac{A_w}{(\theta_1 A_{w1} + \theta_2 A_{w2} + \cdots + \theta_n A_{wn})}, \tag{3.4}$$

where

θ_j is the jth transmission coefficient of material in question; for $i = 1, 2, \ldots, n$, and

A_{wj} is the jth corresponding area of the material in question.

3.6.4   *Rest Period Estimation Formula*

The incorporation of rest periods is essential when humans perform lengthy or strenuous tasks. These periods must be carefully considered during equipment or work design for the effectiveness of human performance. As the length of the rest period may vary from one task to another, the following formula can be used to estimate the length of scheduled or unscheduled rest periods[17]:

$$T_r = T_w \frac{AC - SC}{AC - ARL}, \tag{3.5}$$

where

T_r is the required rest period in minutes,

ARL   is the approximate resting level expressed in kilocalories per minute. The value of ARL is taken as 1.5,

T_w is the working time in minutes,

SC   is the kilocalories per minute adopted as standard, and

AC   is the average energy cost or expenditure expressed in kilocalories per minute of work.

The average energy expenditure in kilocalories per minute and the human heart rate in beats per minute (in parentheses) for tasks such as unloading coal cars in power plants, cleaning floors and tables, packing on conveyors, and bagging and packing paper rolls are: 8 (150), 4.5 (112), 3.7 (113), and 2.5 (113), respectively.

Example 3.3   A professional is performing a certain health care-related task for 140 minutes and his/her average energy expenditure is estimated to be 3 kilocalories per minute. Compute the length of the required rest period if SC = 2.5 kilocalories per minute.

Substituting the given data into Eq. 3.5 yields:

$$T_r = 140 \frac{3 - 2.5}{3 - 1.5}$$

$$\cong 47 \text{ minutes.}$$

This means that the length of the rest period should be around 47 minutes.

3.6.5   *Glare Constant Estimation Formula*

Human errors in health care facilities can occur due to glare. The following formula can be used to estimate the value of the glare constant[17]:

$$K_g = (A)^{0.8} \frac{(LS)^{1.6}}{L_g A_b^2}, \qquad (3.6)$$

where

K_g is the glare constant,
LS   is the luminance of the source,
L_g is the general background luminance,
A_b^2 is the angle between the viewing direction and the direction of the glare source, and
A is the solid angle subtended at the eye by the source.

3.7   Human Factors Checklist and Guidelines

Over the years, human factors professionals have developed a checklist consisting of questions to be addressed to incorporate human factors into the designs of engineering systems. These questions can be specifically tailored to suit an individual situation under consideration. Some examples of these questions are as follows[18]:

- Was adequate attention given to training and complementing work aids?
- Is it easy to identify each and every control device?
- Were the human factor principles considered in the workspace design?
- Were all visual display arrangements optimized?

- Were all controls designed by considering factors such as size, shape, and accessibility?
- Were human decision-making and adaptive capabilities used effectively in the design?
- Are the displays compatible with their corresponding control devices in regard to human factors?
- What type of sensory channels would be the most appropriate for messages to be sent through the displays?
- Were environmental factors such as temperature, illumination, and noise considered with respect to satisfactory levels of human performance?

Nonetheless, some of the important general human factors guidelines for product/system design are as follows:

- Develop a human factors checklist for use during design and production cycle.
- Review the product/system mission/objective with respect to human factors.
- Obtain applicable human factors-related design guide and reference documents.
- Use mockups to "test" the effectiveness of all user-hardware interface designs.
- Utilize the services of human factors specialists as considered appropriate.
- Assemble a hardware prototype (if possible) and evaluate this as much as possible under real-life environments.
- Review with care the final production drawings with respect to human factors.[8]

3.8   Human Factors-Related Data Sources and Useful Publications on Human Factors Data

Various types of human factors-related data are used in the analyses of engineering designs. This includes body dimensions and weights, permissible noise exposure per unit time, human error rates, and energy expenditure per grade of work. Some of the forms in which these data may exist are: expert judgments, design standards, quantitative data tables, mathematical functions and expressions, experience and common sense, and graphic representations.

Some of the important sources for collecting human factors-related data are shown in Fig. 3.2[15]:

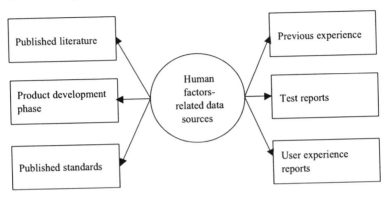

Fig. 3.2.   Important sources for obtaining human factors related data.

The previous experience-related data are obtained from the past similar cases. The published literature is another good source for obtaining human factors-related data and it includes books, reports, journals, and conference proceedings. Various types of human factors-related data can also be obtained during the product development phase. Test reports contain results of tests performed on the manufactured goods.

Published standards are developed by organizations such as professional societies and government agencies and they could be a good source for obtaining various types human factors-related data. The user experience reports contain information on the users' experiences with products.

3.8.1   *Useful Publications on Human Factors Data*

Over the years, many publications containing various types of human factors-related data have appeared. Some of those are listed below:

- Parker, J.F. and West, W.R. (eds), *Bioastronautics Data Book*, Report No. NASA-SP-3006, US Government Printing Office, Washington, D.C.
- *Lighting Handbook*, Prepared by the Illumination Engineering Society, New York, 1971.
- Woodson, W.E., *Human Factors Design Handbook*, McGraw-Hill Book Company, New York, 1981.
- Dhillon, B.S., *Human Reliability with Human Factors*, Pergamon Press, Inc., New York, 1986.

- White, R.M., "The Anthropometry of United States Army Men and Women: 1946–1977," *Human Factors*, Vol. 21, 1979, pp. 473–482.
- Meister, D. and Sullivan, D., *Guide to Human Engineering Design for Visual Displays*, Report No. AD 693-237, 1969, Available from the National Technical Information Service (NTIS), Springfield, Virginia, USA.
- *Anthropometry for Designers, Anthropometrics Source Book 1*, Report No. 1024, National Aeronautic and Space Administration, Washington, D.C., 1978.
- Swain, A. and Guttmann, H., *Handbook of Human Reliability Analysis with Emphasis on Nuclear Power Plant Applications*, Nuclear Regulatory Commission, Washington, D.C., 1980.

Problems

1. What are the three basic categories of man-machine systems? Discuss them in detail.
2. Make a comparison of human and machine capabilities and limitations.
3. List at least six important typical human behaviors.
4. Discuss the following two capabilities of humans:

   - Sight
   - Touch

5. Write an essay on human body measurements.
6. Assume that a meter at a control panel has to be read at the distance of 48 inches and the standard character height at a viewing distance of 28 inches is 0.25. Compute the height of numerals for the specified viewing distance.
7. Write down at least eight important questions for inclusion in a human factor checklist.
8. What are the important sources for obtaining human factors-related data?
9. List at least five documents useful for obtaining human factors data.
10. A health care professional is performing a certain task for 120 minutes and his/her average energy expenditure is estimated to be 2.5 kilocalories per minute. Calculate the length of the required rest period by using Eq. 3.5, if SC = 2 kilocalories per minute.

References

1. Chapanis, A., *Man-Machine Engineering*, Wadsworth Publishing Company, Inc., Belmont, California, 1965.
2. Gilbreth, F.B., *Bricklaying System*, Published by Mryon C. Clark, New York, 1909.
3. Dale Huchingson, R., *New Horizons for Human Factors in Design*, McGraw-Hill Book Company, New York, 1981.
4. Meister, D. and Rabideau, G.F., *Human Factors Evaluation in System Development*, John Wiley and Sons, New York, 1965.
5. Hertzberg, H.T.E., *et al.*, *Anthropometry of Flying Personnel – 1950*, Report No. 53-321 (USAF), Department of Defense, Washington, D.C., 1954.
6. MIL-H-46855, *Human Engineering Requirements for Military Systems, Equipment, and Facilities*, Department of Defense, Washington, D.C., May 1972.
7. McCormick, E.J. and Sanders, M.S., *Human Factors in Engineering and Design*, McGraw Hill Book Company, New York, 1982.
8. Dhillon, B.S., *Advanced Design Concepts for Engineers*, Technomic Publishing Company, Lancaster, Pennsylvania, 1998.
9. Woodson, W.E., *Human Factors Design Handbook*, McGraw Hill Book Company, New York, 1981.
10. AMCP 706-134, *Engineering Design Handbook: Maintainability Guide for Design*, Prepared by the United States Army Material Command, 5001 Eisenhower Avenue, Alexandria, Virginia, 1972.
11. AMCP 706-133, *Engineering Design Handbook: Maintainability Engineering Theory and Practice*, Prepared by the United States Army Material Command, 5001 Eisenhower Avenue, Alexandria, Virginia, 1976.
12. Lederman, S., "Heightening Tactile Impression of Surface Texture," in *Active Touch*, edited by Gordon, G. Pergamon Press, New York, 1978, pp. 40–45.
13. Altman, J.W., *et al.*, *Guide to Design to Mechanical Equipment for Maintainability*, Report No. ASD-TR-61-381, Air Force Systems Command, Wright-Patterson Air Force Base, Ohio, 1961.
14. MIL-STD-1472 (−), *Human Engineering Design Criteria for Military Systems, Equipment, and Facilities*, Department of Defense, Washington, D.C.
15. Peters, G.A. and Adams, B.B., "Three Criteria for Readable Panel Markings," *Product Engineering*, Vol. 30, No. 21, 1959, pp. 55–57.
16. Dale Huchingson, R., *New Horizons for Human Factors in Design*, McGraw Hill Book Company, New York, 1981.
17. Oborne, D.J., *Ergonomics at Work*, John Wiley and Sons, New York, 1982.
18. Dhillon, B.S., *Engineering Design: A Modern Approach*, Richard D. Irwin, Inc., Chicago, 1996.

Chapter 4

Human Reliability and Error Basics

4.1 Introduction

Although human reliability and error may mean basically the same thing to many people, but from time to time their distinction can be quite important. Their fundamental difference is conveyed by their definitions as follows. Human reliability is defined as the probability that a task will be accomplished successfully by an individual at any required stage in a system operation within a specified minimum time (i.e. if the time requirement exists).[1,2] Similarly, human error is defined as a failure to carry out a specified job/task (or the performance of a prohibited action), which could result in the damage to properties or the disruption of scheduled operations.[2,3]

The history of the philosophy on human reliability and error may be traced back to the late 1950s when H.L. Williams pointed out that human-element reliability must be included in the system-reliability prediction; otherwise the predicted value would not represent the real system-reliability picture.[4] A study conducted in 1960 revealed that human error is responsible for 20 to 50% of all equipment failures.[5] In 1973, IEEE Transactions on Reliability, a well-known journal in the field of reliability, published a special issue devoted to human reliability.[6] The first commercially available book on human reliability appeared in 1986.[7]

Over the years, a vast number of publications on human reliability and error have appeared.[8–10] This chapter presents the various fundamental aspects of human reliability and error.

4.2   Human Performance Characteristics, Occupational Stressors, General Stress Factors, and Human Operator Stress Characteristics

Stress is an important factor that affects human performance and reliability. Obviously, an overstressed individual will have a higher probability of making mistakes. Over the years various researchers have studied the relationship between human performance effectiveness and anxiety or stress and have concluded the human performance effectiveness versus stress relationship as shown in Fig. 4.1.[11–12] The figure depicts that stress to a moderate level is essential in achieving optimal human performance effectiveness. Otherwise, at very low stress levels, the task will be dull and unchallenging, thus human performance will not be at its maximum value.

In contrast, stress beyond a moderate level will lead to the deterioration in human performance. Some of the reasons for performance deterioration are worry, fear, or other kinds of psychological stress. Nonetheless, moderate stress may simply be described as the level of stress sufficient to keep the individual alert. All in all, it may be concluded that the probability of human error occurrence is greater under high stress than under moderate stress.

There are four types of occupational stressors as shown in Fig. 4.2: workload-related, occupational frustration-related, occupational change-related, and miscellaneous.[11]

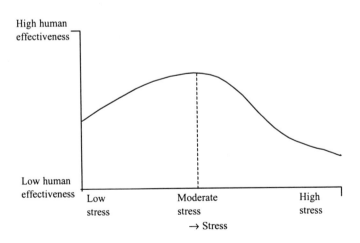

Fig. 4.1.   Human performance effectiveness versus stress curve.

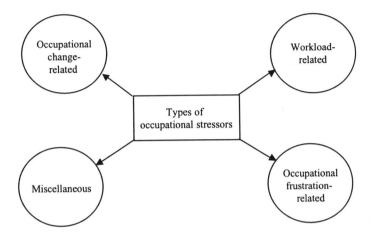

Fig. 4.2. Classifications of occupational stressors.

The workload-related stressors are concerned with work overload or work underload. In the case of work overload the job or position requirements exceed the person's ability to satisfy them effectively. On the other hand, in the case of work underload, the current functions being performed by the individual provide insufficient stimulation. Examples of work underload include task repetitiveness, the lack of opportunity to utilize the individual's acquired expertise and skills, and the lack of any intellectual input.

The occupational frustration-related stressors are concerned with the problems of occupational frustration. More specifically, the conditions where the job inhibits the meeting of set goals. Some examples of occupational frustration-related problems are: the lack of proper communication, the ambiguity of one's role, poor career development guidance, and bureaucracy difficulties.

The occupational change-related stressors are concerned with factors that disrupt the individual's behavioral, cognitive, and physiological patterns of functioning. Usually, this type of stressors exists in organizations concerned with growth and productivity. Examples of occupational changes include promotion, relocation, scientific developments, and organizational restructuring.

The miscellaneous stressors incorporate all other stressors that are not included in the above three classifications. Some examples of these stressors are: too little or too much lighting, noise, and poor interpersonal relationships.

Past experiences indicate that there are many general factors that increase stress on an individual; thus leading to a decrease in his/her reliability. These factors include the possibility of redundancy at work, serious financial difficulties, unhappiness with the current job, having to work with individuals with unpredictable temperaments, excessive demands from superiors at work, poor health, working under extremely tight time pressures, poor chances for promotion, experiencing difficulties with spouse or children or both, and lacking the expertise to perform the ongoing job.[8]

In performing a given task, the human operator may have certain limitations. When these limitations are violated, the error occurrence probability increases.[1] This probability can be reduced quite significantly if the operator limitations or characteristics are considered with care during the design phase. Nonetheless, some of the operator stress characteristics are as follows:

- Having a very short decision-making time.
- Making a quick comparison of two or more displays.
- The performance of task requiring a very long sequence of steps.
- Requirement to perform task steps at high speed.
- Difficulty in discriminating more than one display.
- Requirement for making decisions on the basis of data obtained from various different sources.
- Inadequate feedback information to determine the correctness of actions taken.
- Requirement to operate two or more controls simultaneously at high speed.
- The requirement for prolonged monitoring.

4.3   Human Performance Reliability and Correctability Functions

4.3.1   *Human Performance Reliability Function*

From time to time humans perform various types of time-continuous tasks: scope monitoring, aircraft maneuvering, missile countdown, etc. In situations such as these, human performance reliability is an important parameter. A general human performance reliability function for time-continuous tasks can be developed in the same manner as the development of the reliability function for hardware systems. Thus, we write[13]:

$$\lambda_h(t) = -\frac{1}{R_h(t)} \cdot \frac{dR_h(t)}{dt},$$ (4.1)

where

t is time,

$\lambda_h(t)$ is the human hazard rate or time dependent error rate, and

$R_h(t)$ is the human performance reliability at time t.

By rearranging Eq. 4.1, we get:

$$\frac{1}{R_h(t)} \cdot dR_h(t) = -\lambda_h(t)\, dt.$$ (4.2)

Integrating both sides of Eq. 4.2 over the time interval $[0, t]$, we write:

$$\int_1^{R_h(t)} \frac{1}{R_h(t)} dR_h(t) = -\int_0^t \lambda_h(t)\, dt,$$ (4.3)

since at $t = 0$, $R_h(t) = 1$.

After evaluating the left-hand side of Eq. 4.3, we obtain:

$$\ln R_h(t) = -\int_0^t \lambda_h(t)\, dt.$$ (4.4)

Thus, from Eq. 4.4, we obtain:

$$R_h(t) = e^{-\int_0^t \lambda_h(t)\, dt}.$$ (4.5)

The above expression is applicable in all circumstances, irrespective of the human error rate being constant or nonconstant, and more specifically, irrespective of the times to human error which is defined by statistical distributions such as exponential, Weibull, or normal. Nonetheless, an experimental study, concerning time continuous vigilance tasks, was performed.[14] In this study, the subjects were asked to observe a clock-type display of lights and when a light failed they responded to it by pressing a hand-held switch. The data collected from this study was used miss errors, i.e. when the subjects failed to detect the failed lights. Statistical distributions such as the Weibull, gamma, and the lognormal fitted quite well to various types of data collected from this study.[14]

By integrating Eq. 4.5 over the time interval $[0, \infty]$, we obtain:

$$\text{MTTHE} = \int_0^\infty \left[e^{- \int_0^t \lambda_h(t)\, dt} \right] dt, \qquad (4.6)$$

where MTTHE is the mean time to human error.

Example 4.1   A healthcare professional is performing some time continuous task and his/her error rate is $\lambda_h(t) = \lambda_h = 0.002$ error/hour. Calculate the professional's reliability for an 8-hour mission and the mean time to human error.

By substituting the given data into Eq. 4.5, we get:

$$R_h(8) = e^{- \int_0^8 (0.002)\, dt}$$

$$= e^{-(0.002)(8)}$$

$$= 0.9841.$$

Using the given human error rate value in Eq. 4.6, we obtain:

$$\text{MTTHE} = \int_0^\infty \left[e^{- \int_0^t (0.002)\, dt} \right] dt$$

$$= \int_0^\infty e^{-(0.002)t}\, dt$$

$$= \frac{1}{0.002}$$

$$= 500 \text{ hours}.$$

Thus the healthcare professional's reliability for an 8-hour mission and the mean time to human error are 0.9841 and 500 hours, respectively.

4.3.2   *Human Performance Correctability Function*

This may simply be described as the probability that an error will be corrected in time t subjected to task associated stress constraints and environments. Mathematically, the human performance correctability function is expressed by[14]:

$$PC(t) = 1 - e^{- \int_0^t ec(t)\, dt}, \qquad (4.7)$$

where

$PC(t)$ is the probability that an error will be corrected in time t, and
$ec(t)$ is the time t dependent rate at which tasks are corrected.

Equation 4.7 holds for any time-to-correction statistical distribution, for example, the exponential, normal, Rayleigh, or the Weibull distribution.

Alternatively, the human performance correctability function may be defined as follows:

$$PC(t) = \int_0^t f_c(t)\, dt, \tag{4.8}$$

where $f_c(t)$ is the time-to-correction completion probability density function.

Example 4.2   Assume that a healthcare professional is performing a certain task and his/her error correction rate is $ec(t) = ec$ and the times-to-error correction are exponentially distributed, i.e.

$$f_c(t) = ece^{-ect}. \tag{4.9}$$

Obtain expressions for the professional's correctability function by using Eqs. 4.7 and 4.8. Comment on the resulting expressions.

Using the given expressions in Eqs. 4.7 and 4.8, we obtain:

$$PC(t) = 1 - e^{-\int_0^t ec\, dt}$$
$$= 1 - e^{-ect}, \text{ and} \tag{4.10}$$
$$PC(t) = \int_0^t ece^{-ect}\, dt$$
$$= 1 - e^{-ect}. \tag{4.11}$$

Equations 4.10 and 4.11 are identical.

Example 4.3   A healthcare professional's error correction rate is 0.4 error/hour. Calculate the probability that an error will be corrected by the professional during a 6-hour mission, by using Eq. 4.11.

By inserting the given data into Eq. 4.11, we get

$$PC(6) = 1 - e^{-(0.4)(6)}$$
$$= 0.9093.$$

There is an approximately 91% probability that the healthcare professional will correct an error during the specified time period.

4.4   Human Reliability Analysis Methods

Over the years many human reliability analysis methods have been developed.[7] This section presents some specific human analysis methods. The more general ones are presented in Chapter 5.

4.4.1   *The Throughput Ratio Method*

This method is used to determine the operability of man-machine interfaces/stations and was developed by the US Navy Electronics Laboratory Center.[15] The operability may be defined as the extent to which the man-machine station performance meets the design expectation for the station under consideration.

The term "throughput" basically means transmission, because the ratio is in terms of responses per unit time emitted by the human operator. Nonetheless, the throughput ratio in percentage is expressed as follows[15]:

$$\text{MMO} = \left[\frac{\theta_1}{\theta_2} - \text{CF} \right] (100), \qquad (4.12)$$

where

MMO   is the man-machine operability or the throughput ratio in percentage,

CF   is the correction factor,

θ_1 is the number of throughput items generated or performed per unit time, and

θ_2 is the number of throughput items to be generated or performed per unit time in order to meet design expectations.

In turn, the correction factor is expressed by:

$$\text{CF} = A_1 A_2, \qquad (4.13)$$

$$A_1 = \frac{\alpha_1}{\alpha_2} \left(\frac{\theta_1}{\theta_2} \right), \text{ and} \qquad (4.14)$$

$$A_2 = A_1 P_e^2 P_f, \qquad (4.15)$$

where

α_1 is the number of trials in which the control-display operation is performed incorrectly,

α_2 is the total number of trials in which the control-display operation is performed,

P_e is the probability that the human operator will not detect the error, and

P_f is the probability of function failure due to human error.

The throughput ratio method can be used for various purposes such as to rectify human factor discrepancies, to demonstrate system acceptability, to compare alternative design operabilities, and to establish the feasibility of systems.

Example 4.4   Assume that we have the following data for a certain medical system:

- $P_e = 0.25$
- $P_f = 0.55$
- $\theta_1 = 5$
- $\theta_2 = 10$
- $\alpha_1 = 4$
- $\alpha_2 = 12$

Calculate the value of the throughput ratio. By substituting the above given values into Eqs. 4.12–4.15, we get:

$$A_1 = \frac{4}{12}\left(\frac{5}{10}\right) = 0.1667,$$

$$A_2 = (0.1667)(0.25)^2(0.55)$$

$$= 0.0057,$$

$$CF = (0.1667)(0.0057)$$

$$= 0.001, \text{ and}$$

$$MMO = \left[\frac{5}{10} - 0.001\right](100)$$

$$= 49.90\%.$$

Thus the value of the man-machine operability or throughput ratio is 49.90%.

4.4.2   *Pontecorvo Method*

This method can be used to obtain reliability estimates of task performance. More specifically, the method is concerned with obtaining reliability estimates of discrete and separate subtasks having no accurate reliability figures. These estimates are combined to obtain the overall task reliability estimate. The method is used during the initial design phases to quantitatively assess the interaction of men and machines. Furthermore, the technique is also quite useful in determining the performance of an individual acting alone.

Nonetheless, the Pontecorvo approach is composed of the following six steps[16]:

- **Identify tasks.** This is concerned with the identification of tasks to be performed. These tasks are usually identified at a gross level. It simply means that each task represents one complete operation.
- **Identify task components.** This is concerned with identifying each task's subtasks. More specifically, the subtasks that are essential to complete the task.
- **Collect empirical performance data.** This is concerned with obtaining relevant empirical performance data subjected to environments under which the subtask is to be performed.
- **Establish subtask rate.** This is concerned with rating each subtask with respect to the potential for error or the difficulty level. Usually, a 10-point scale is used in judging the subtask rate, e.g. 1 for the least likelihood of error and 10 for the most likelihood of error.
- **Express data in the form of a regression equation.** This is basically concerned with predicting the subtask reliability. The subtask reliability is predicted by expressing the empirical data and judging the data ratings in the form of a straight line and then testing it (i.e. the line) for the goodness-of-fit.
- **Estimate task reliability.** This is concerned with determining the task reliability. The task reliability is estimated by multiplying the subtask reliabilities.

All in all, the above six steps are used to determine the performance reliability of an individual acting alone. However, the availability of a backup individual helps to improve the probability of the task being performed correctly. Past experiences indicate that from time to time a backup person may be available for a certain amount of time but not all the time. Under such scenario, the overall reliability of two individuals working together to accomplish a task is given by:

$$R_T = \frac{\{1 - (1 - R_S)^2\}P_a + R_S P_u}{P_a + P_u}, \tag{4.16}$$

where

R_T is the overall reliability of two individuals working together to accomplish a task,

R_S is the reliability of the single individual,

P_a is the percentage of time the backup individual is available, and

P_u is the percentage of time the backup individual is unavailable.

Example 4.5   Assume that two independent professionals are working together to perform a healthcare task. As per previous experiences, the reliability of each professional is 0.90 and the backup professional is available only for 85% of the time. In other words, for 15% of the time the backup individual is not available. Calculate the probability of performing the healthcare task correctly.

By substituting the given data values into Eq. 4.16, we obtain:

$$R_T = \frac{\{1 - (1 - 0.9)^2\}0.85 + (0.9)(0.15)}{0.85 + 0.15}$$

$$= 0.9765.$$

It means that the probability of performing the healthcare task correctly is 97.65%.

4.4.3   *Personnel Reliability Index Method*

This index method was developed by the United States Navy to provide feedback on the technical proficiency of the electronic maintenance manpower and it is based on the following nine job factors[17]:

- Equipment operation
- Instructions
- Equipment inspection
- Personnel relationships
- Electronic circuit analysis
- Electro repair
- Using reference materials
- Electro safety
- Electro cognition

Various types of activities are associated with the above factors. Some of the activities pertaining to electro safety, electro repair, instructions, personnel relationship, equipment operation, and equipment inspection are cited as follows:

- Supervising and inspecting electronic equipment.
- Repairing equipment in the shop.
- Operating equipment.
- Teaching other people with respect to maintenance.
- Making use of safety precautions on oneself and on equipment.
- Operating electrical and electronics test equipment.

Some activities pertaining specifically to using-reference-materials, electro cognition, and electronic circuit analysis are presented in Table 4.1.

In the Navy, data was collected from maintenance supervisors for each of the above nine factors over a period of two months. These data are basically concerned with the number of uncommonly effective and ineffective performances by people involved with the maintenance activity. For each job factor, the following index, R, is calculated by using these data:

$$R = \frac{\sum \text{EB}}{\sum \text{EB} + \sum \text{IB}}, \qquad (4.17)$$

where

EB   are the uncommonly effective behaviors, and
IB   are the uncommonly ineffective behaviors.

The value of the index R varies between 0 and 1 and the overall effectiveness, R_0, for a maintenance person is calculated by using the following equation:

$$R_o = \prod_{i=1}^{9} R_i, \qquad (4.18)$$

Table 4.1.   Activities pertaining to three different job factors.

No.	Job Factor	Activities
1	Using-reference-materials	• Interpreting reports • Using supporting reference materials
2	Electro cognition	• Maintenance and troubleshooting of electronic equipment • Use of electronic maintenance reference material
3	Electronic circuit analysis	• Preparing failure reports • Keeping maintenance usage data • Understanding electronic circuitry principles

where R_i is the index value (i.e. reliability) of job factor i; for $i = 1, 2, \ldots, 9$.

Two important anticipated uses of this index are design analysis as well as manpower selection and training. All in all, with some proper tailoring, it can also be used in the healthcare area.

4.5 Human Error Occurrence Reasons and Its Consequences

In general, it may be said that most human errors occur because humans are capable of doing so many different things in varying ways and manners. Nonetheless, some of the important and specific reasons for the occurrence of human errors are as follows[18]:

- Poor equipment design and poorly written equipment maintenance and operating procedures.
- Inadequate training to people such as operating, maintenance, and production workers.
- Inadequate lighting in the work area.
- Poor work layout and crowded workspace.
- Improper work tools and inadequate equipment handling.
- Complex task and poor motivation.
- High noise and temperature in the work area.
- Poor verbal communication.
- Poor management.

The consequences of a human error may vary from one situation to another, from one piece of equipment to another, or from one task to another. Moreover, consequences may range from minor to very severe, for example, from minor delays in system performance to a major loss of lives. Nonetheless, with respect to equipment, the consequences of a human error may be classified under the following categories[18]:

- **Category A:** Equipment operation is stopped completely.
- **Category B:** Equipment operation is delayed quite significantly but not stopped totally.
- **Category C:** Delay in equipment operation is insignificant.

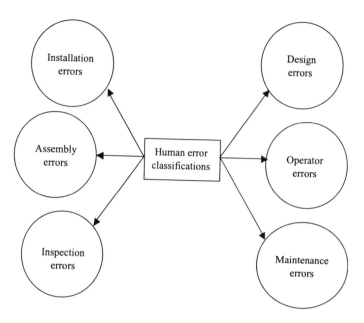

Fig. 4.3.   Six classifications of human errors.

4.6   Human Error Occurrence Ways and Classification

Over the years professionals working in the field of human factors have identified various ways in which a human error can occur. The five commonly accepted ways are as follows[19]:

- **Way I:** Failure to perform a required function.
- **Way II:** Failure to recognize a hazardous condition.
- **Way III:** Making a wrong decision in response to a problem.
- **Way IV:** Poor timing and inadequate response to a contingency.
- **Way V:** Performing a task that should not be accomplished.

Human errors may be categorized under various classifications. Figure 4.3 presents the six commonly used classifications.[18,20]

4.7   Human Error Analysis Models

In the published literature, there are many mathematical models that can be used to perform various types of human error analysis. This section presents two such models.

4.7.1 *Model I*

This model can be used to determine the accuracy of a quality inspector and it was originally developed by J.M. Juran in 1935.[21] The model is based on the assumption that the inspectors involved with quality control work can accept bad items and reject good ones. In addition, check inspectors are present to re-examine the output of regular inspectors. Thus, the reliability or the accuracy of an inspector in percentage is expressed by:

$$RA = \frac{(\beta - G)(100)}{(\beta - G + DM)},$$ (4.19)

where

RA is the inspector reliability or accuracy. More specifically, the percentage of defects correctly identified by the regular inspector,

β is the number of defects discovered by the regular inspector,

DM is the total number of defects missed by the regular inspector, and

G is the total number of good items rejected by the regular inspector.

Example 4.6 A healthcare professional inspected a lot of medical items and found 75 defects. Subsequently, another healthcare professional re-examined the entire lot and found that the first healthcare professional missed 25 defects and rejected 5 good items. Calculate the reliability or accuracy of the first professional.

By substituting the given data into Eq. 4.19, we obtain:

$$RA = \frac{(75 - 5)(100)}{(75 - 5 + 25)}$$
$$= 73.68\%.$$

Thus, the reliability or accuracy of the first healthcare professional is 73.68%.

4.7.2 *Model II*

This model is concerned with determining the reliability of a parallel system with critical and non-critical human errors. The system is subjected to the following assumptions[7]:

- All system units are independent and active.

- At least one unit must operate normally for the system success.
- Each unit failures can be grouped under two categories: hardware failures and human errors.
- The system fails when all of its units fail.

The human errors associated with the system are classified under two categories: critical and non-critical. The occurrence of a critical human error causes the failure of the complete system. In contrast, the occurrence of a non-critical human error causes only a single unit to fail.

Figure 4.4 shows a block diagram of the model. The parallel system is composed of m units. In turn, each unit has two hypothetical elements: one representing unit hardware failures and the other representing unit human errors or non-critical human errors. A hypothetical unit representing all critical human errors is connected in series with the parallel system.

The reliability, R_S, of the non-identical unit system as shown in Fig. 4.4 is given by:

$$R_S = \left[1 - \prod_{i=1}^{m} \{1 - (1 - F_i)(1 - H_i)\} \right] (1 - H_C), \qquad (4.20)$$

where

  m is the total number of active units,
  H_C is the failure probability of the parallel system due to critical human error,

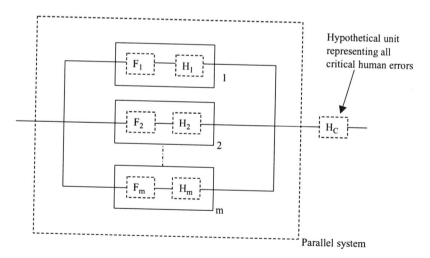

Fig. 4.4.   Block diagram of a parallel system with critical and non-critical human errors.

H_i is the failure probability of unit i due to non-critical human error, for $i = 1, 2, 3, \ldots, m$, and

F_i is the hardware failure probability of unit i, for $i = 1, 2, 3, \ldots, m$.

For identical units, Eq. 4.20 simplifies to:

$$R_S = [1 - \{1 - (1 - F)(1 - H)\}^m](1 - H_C), \qquad (4.21)$$

where

F is the unit hardware failure probability, and

H is the unit failure probability due to non-critical human error.

For exponentially distributed hardware failures, critical human errors, and non-critical human errors, the cumulative distribution functions, respectively, are[2]:

$$F(t) = \int_0^t \lambda_F e^{-\lambda_F t} \, dt$$

$$= 1 - e^{-\lambda_F t}, \qquad (4.22)$$

$$H_C(t) = \int_0^t \lambda_{Hc} e^{-\lambda_{Hc} t} \, dt$$

$$= 1 - e^{-\lambda_{Hc} t}, \text{ and} \qquad (4.23)$$

$$H(t) = \int_0^t \lambda_H e^{-\lambda_H t} \, dt$$

$$= 1 - e^{-\lambda_H t}, \qquad (4.24)$$

where

λ_F is the unit hardware failure rate,

λ_{Hc} is the critical human error rate,

λ_H is the non-critical human error rate,

$F(t)$ is the unit hardware failure probability at time t,

$H_c(t)$ is the system failure probability due to critical human error at time t, and

$H(t)$ is the unit failure probability due to non-critical human error at time t.

By substituting Eqs. 4.22–4.24 into Eq. 4.21, we get:

$$R_S(t) = [1 - \{1 - e^{-(\lambda_F + \lambda_H)t}\}^m]e^{-\lambda_{Hc} t}, \qquad (4.25)$$

where $R_S(t)$ is the reliability of the identical unit parallel system with critical and non-critical human errors at time t.

Integrating Eq. 4.25 over the time interval $[0, \infty]$, we get:

$$\text{MTTF}_S = \int_0^\infty [1 - \{1 - e^{-(\lambda_F + \lambda_H)t}\}^m]e^{-\lambda_{HC}t}\, dt$$

$$= \frac{1}{\lambda_{Hc}} - \sum_{i=0}^{m} \binom{m}{i}(-1)^{m-i}\frac{1}{(m-i)(\lambda_F + \lambda_H) + \lambda_{Hc}}, \qquad (4.26)$$

where

$$\binom{m}{i} \equiv \frac{m!}{(m-i)!i!}, \text{ and}$$

MTTF$_S$ is the mean time to failure of parallel systems with critical and non-critical human errors.

Example 4.7   A medical system is composed of two independent, identical, and active units in parallel. The system is subjected to critical and non-critical human error. More specifically, the occurrence of a critical human error causes system failure and, on the other hand, the occurrence of a non-critical human error only causes an unit failure. The critical and non-critical human error rates are 0.0001 errors/hour and 0.008 errors/hour, respectively. In addition, the failure rate of a unit is 0.009 failures/hour.

Calculate the medical system mean time to failure and the reliability for a 50-hour mission.

By inserting the given data into Eq. 4.25, we get:

$$R_S(50) = [1 - \{1 - e^{-(0.009+0.008)(50)}\}^2]e^{-(0.0001)(50)}$$
$$= (1 - 0.3279)(0.9950)$$
$$= 0.6688.$$

Similarly, by substituting the specified data values into Eq. 4.26, we get:

$$\text{MTTF}_S = \frac{1}{0.001} - \sum_{i=0}^{2} \binom{2}{i}(-1)^{2-i}\frac{1}{(2-i)(0.009+0.008)+0.0001}$$

$$= \frac{1}{0.0001} - \left[\frac{1}{2(0.009+0.008)+0.0001}\right.$$

$$\left. -\frac{2}{(0.009+0.008+0.0001)} + \frac{1}{0.0001}\right]$$

$$= 87.63 \text{ hours.}$$

The medical system reliability and the mean time to failure are 0.6688 and 87.63 hours, respectively.

Problems

1. Write an essay on the history of human reliability.
2. Discuss human performance characteristics and occupational stressors.
3. List at least nine human operator stress characteristics.
4. Prove that human reliability, $R_h(t)$, is given by:

$$R_h(t) = e^{-\int_0^t \lambda_h(t)\, dt}, \tag{4.27}$$

   where $\lambda_h(t)$ is the human time (t) dependent error rate.
5. Assume that a healthcare professional is performing a certain time continuous task and his/her error rate is 0.004 error/hour. Compute the professional's reliability for a 5-hour mission and the mean time to human error.
6. Define human performance correctability function.
7. Discuss the following human reliability analysis methods:

   - The throughput ratio method
   - The Pontecorvo method

8. List at least ten important reasons for the occurrence of human errors.
9. Discuss the ways in which a human error can occur.
10. A healthcare professional inspected a lot of medical items and discovered 50 defects. Subsequently, another healthcare professional re-examined the entire lot and found that his/her predecessor missed 15 defects and rejected 3 good items. Compute the reliability or accuracy of the first professional.

References

1. Meister, D., "Human Factors in Reliability," in *Reliability Handbook*, edited by W.G. Ireson, McGraw Hill Book Company, New York, 1966, pp. 400–415.
2. Dhillon, B.S. and Singh, C., *Engineering Reliability: New Techniques and Applications*, John Wiley and Sons, New York, 1981.
3. Hagen, E.W., (ed), "Human Reliability Analysis," *Nuclear Safety*, Vol. 17, 1976, pp. 315–326.
4. Williams, H.L., "Reliability Evaluation of the Human Component in Man-Machine System," *Electrical Manufacturing*, April 1958, pp. 78–82.

5. Shapero, A., Cooper, J.I., Rappaport, M., Shaeffer, K.H., and Bates, C.J., *Human Engineering Testing and Malfunction Data Collection in Weapon System Programs*, WADD Technical Report No. 60–36, Wright-Patterson Air Force Base, Dayton, Ohio, February 1960.

6. Regulinski, T.L., (ed), "Special Issue on Human Reliability," *IEEE Transactions on Reliability*, Vol. 22, August 1973.

7. Dhillon, B.S., *Human Reliability with Human Factors*, Pergamon Press, Inc., New York, 1986.

8. Dhillon, B.S., "On Human Reliability: Bibliography," *Microelectronics and Reliability*, Vol. 20, 1980, pp. 371–373.

9. Lee, K.W., Tillman, F.A., and Higgins, J.J., "A Literature Survey of the Human Reliability, Component in a Man-Machine System," *IEEE Transactions on Reliability*, Vol. 37, 1988, pp. 24–34.

10. Dhillon, B.S. and Yang, N., "Human Reliability: A Literature Survey and Review," *Microelectronics and Reliability*, Vol. 34, 1994, pp. 803–810.

11. Beech, H.R., Burns, L.E., and Sheffield, B.F., *A Behavioral Approach to the Management of Stress*, John Wiley and Sons, New York, 1982.

12. Hagen, E.W., (ed), "Human Reliability Analysis," *Nuclear Safety*, Vol. 17, 1976, pp. 315–326.

13. Shooman, M.L., *Probabilistic Reliability: An Engineering Approach*, McGraw Hill Book Company, New York, 1968.

14. Regulinski, T.L. and Askren, W.B., "Mathematical Modeling of Human Performance Reliability," *Proceedings of the Annual Symposium on Reliability*, 1969, pp. 5–11.

15. Meister, D., *Comparative Analysis of Human Reliability Models*, Report No. AD 734-432, 1971. Available from the National Technical Information Service, Springfield, Virginia, USA.

16. Pontecorvo, A.B., "A Method of Predicting Human Reliability," *Proceedings of the 4th Annual Reliability and Maintainability Conference*, 1965, pp. 337–342. This proceedings was published by Spartan Books, Washington, D.C.

17. Siegel, A.I. and Federman, P.J., *Development of Performance Evaluative Measures*, Report No. 7071-2, Contract No 014-67-00107, Office of Naval Research, United States Navy, Washington, D.C., September 1970.

18. Meister, D., "The Problem of Human-Initiated Failures," *Proceedings of the 8th National Symposium on Reliability and Quality Control*, 1962, pp. 234–239.

19. Hammer, W., *Product Safety Management and Engineering*, Prentice Hall, Englewood Cliffs, New Jersey, 1980.

20. Juran, J.M., "Inspector's Errors in Quality Control," *Mechanical Engineering*, Vol. 57, 1935, pp. 643–644.

Chapter 5

Methods for Performing Human Reliability and Error Analysis in Health Care System

5.1 Introduction

Today, the fields of reliability, safety, quality, and human factors are well-established disciplines. Over the years, a large volume of published literature in each of these areas has appeared in the form of books, conference proceedings, journal articles, and technical reports. Many new concepts and techniques have been developed in these areas. Some of the methods and techniques developed in these areas are being used across many diverse disciplines including engineering design, production, maintenance, and management.

One example is the fault tree analysis (FTA), developed in reliability engineering, which is being used in performing design, production, maintenance, and management studies.

Another example of a widely used method across diverse disciplines is the failure mode and effects analysis (FMEA). Originally this technique was developed for application in the field of reliability engineering. Needless to say, there are a large number of methods and techniques developed the subject of reliability, safety, quality, and human factors, that are applied in various other areas. Therefore, this chapter presents a number of useful methods and techniques for performing human reliability and error analysis in health care system extracted from areas such as those mentioned above.

5.2   Failure Modes and Effect Analysis (FMEA)

This is a widely used method in many industries for the analysis of engineering systems from reliability and safety aspects. FMEA may simply be described as a powerful approach used to conduct the analysis of each potential failure mode in the system under consideration to determine the results or effects of such modes on the entire system.[1] In the event when the method is extended to categorize each potential failure effect according to its severity; it is referred to as the failure mode effects and criticality analysis (FMECA). The method was developed in the early 1950s by the US Navy's Bureau of Aeronautics and it was termed "Failure Analysis".[2] Subsequently, the method was renamed to "Failure Effect Analysis" and the Bureau of Naval Weapons introduced it into its new specification on flight control systems.[3]

In order to ensure the desired reliability of the space systems, National Aeronautics and Space Administration (NASA) extended the functions of the FMEA and renamed it FMECA.[4] In the 1970s, the US Department of Defense developed a military standard entitled "Procedures for Performing a Failure Mode, Effects, and Criticality Analysis".[5]

A comprehensive list of references on FMEA is given in Ref. 6.

The main steps involved in performing FMEA are as follows[4,7]:

- **Define the system and its related needs.** This basically involves breaking down the system into blocks, block functions, and the interface between them. Past experiences indicate that usually in the initial stages of the program a reasonably good system definition does not exist and the analyst involved establishes his/her own system definition with the aid of documents such as drawings, development plans and specifications, and trade study reports.
- **Develop the appropriate ground rules.** These rules are developed as to how the FMEA will be subsequently performed. Once the system definition and the mission requirements are reasonably completed, the development of ground rules becomes quite a straightforward process. Some examples of the ground rules are as follows:
  - Limits of operational and environmental stresses.
  - Statement of primary and secondary mission objectives.
  - Delineation of mission phases.
  - Definition of what constitutes failure of system hardware components.
  - Description of the coding system employed.
  - Statement of analysis level.

- **Describe in detail the system and its functional blocks.** Basically, this step is concerned with the preparation of the system description which can be grouped under two parts:

  - **Part I: System block diagram.** This diagram is used to determine the success/failure relationships among all the system parts. More specifically it graphically shows the system parts to be analyzed, the series and redundant relationships among the parts, the inputs and outputs of the system, and each system part's inputs and outputs.
  - **Part II: Narrative functional statement.** This is developed for the entire system as well as for each subsystem and component. The statement provides a narrative description of each item's operation for each mission phase/operational mode. The degree of the description detail depends on various factors including the uniqueness of the functions performed and the application of the item under consideration.

- **Identify all possible failure modes and their associated effects.** This is basically concerned with performing analysis of the failure modes and their effects; usually by using a well-designed form or a worksheet. The form collects information on many areas including item identification, item function, failure modes and causes, failure effects on system/subsystem/mission/personnel, failure detection method, compensating provisions, criticality classification, and other remarks.

- **Develop a critical items' list.** This is prepared to facilitate the communication of important analysis results to the management and it includes information on areas such as item identification, concise statement of failure mode, degree of loss effect, criticality classification, retention rationale, and the FMEA worksheet page number.

- **Document the analysis.** This step is concerned with the documentation of the analysis and is equivalent in importance to all the previous steps because poor documentation can lead to the ineffectiveness of the FMEA process. The FMEA report includes items such as those listed below:

  - System definition.
  - System description.
  - Ground rules.
  - Failure modes and their effects.
  - Critical items list.

5.2.1   *FMEA Benefits*

Over the years FMEA has been applied in many diverse areas. Some of the benefits observed with the application of this method are as follows[8,9]:

- It is comprehensible.
- It reduces the item development time and cost.
- It improves customer satisfaction.
- It highlights safety concerns to be focused on.
- It improves communication among design interface personnel.
- It reduces engineering changes.
- It is a systematic approach in classifying hardware failures.
- It provides a safeguard against repeating the same mistake in the future.
- It is useful to compare alternative designs.

5.3   Root Cause Analysis (RCA)

This method has been used for many years in the industry and it was originally developed by the United States Department of Energy[10] for the investigation of industrial incidents. RCA may simply be described as a systematic investigation approach that makes use of information collected during an assessment of an accident to determine the underlying factors for the deficiencies that led to the accident.[11]

RCA starts with the outlining of the event sequence leading to the occurrence of the accident. Starting with the adverse event itself, the analyst involved performs his/her functions backwards in time, ascertaining and recording each and every important event. In collecting such information, it is very important for the analyst to avoid making a premature judgment, blame, and attribution, but to focus on the incident facts with care. This way the clearly defined actions leading to an event will help the investigation team to confidently ask a question, "Why did it (event) occur?".[12]

The performance of the RCA helps in understanding better the causal factors in the sequence of evolving events.[13] The RCA process is concluded with recommendations for improvements based on the investigational findings.

In the United States, the Joint Commission on the Accreditation of Healthcare Organizations (JCAHO) recommends that health care facilities should respond to all sentinel events, in an effective manner, within 45 days of their occurrence by using RCA. Moreover, RCA must possess, at least, the following characteristics for its acceptability by the JCAHO[14]:

- The analysis is absolutely thorough and credible.
- The focus of the analysis is basically on systems and processes, not on individual performances.
- The analysis repeatedly probes deeper by simply asking "Why?", and when answered, it will question "Why?" again, etc.
- The analysis systematically progresses from special causes in clinical-related processes to common causes in organizational-related processes.
- The analysis clearly highlights the appropriate changes that can be made in processes and systems by either redesigning or developing new systems/processes that would definitely lower the risk of the occurrence of sentinel events in the future.

General steps to perform RCA in healthcare are as follows[15]:

- Educate all concerned about RCA.
- Inform all appropriate staff when the occurrence of a sentinel event is reported.
- Form an RCA team by including all appropriate individuals.
- Prepare for and conduct the first team meeting.
- Determine the event sequence.
- Separate and identify each event sequence that may have been a contributory factor in the occurrence of the sentinel event.
- Seriously brainstorm about the factors surrounding the chosen events that may have been, direct or indirect, contributory to the occurrence of the sentinel event.
- Affinitize with the results of the brainstorming session.
- Prepare the action plan.
- Distribute the RCA document and the associated action plan to all people concerned.

5.3.1   *RCA Softwares*

Over the years various types of software packages have been developed to perform the RCA. Some of the advantages cited for the automation of RCA are the reduction in analysis time, better data organization, easier reporting capabilities, improved rigor, and enhanced follow-up capabilities.[11]

Some of the available RCA software packages in the market are presented in Table 5.1.[11]

Table 5.1.   RCA software packages.

No.	Package Name	Developed by
1	BRAVO	JBF Associates, Inc.
		1000 Technology Drive
		Knoxville, TN 37939, USA
2	PROACT	Reliability Center, Inc.
		P.O. Box 1421
		Hopewell, VA 23860, USA
3	TAPROOT	System Improvements, Inc.
		238 S. Peters Road, Suite 301
		Knoxville, TN 37923-5224, USA
4	REASON	Decision Systems, Inc.
		802 N. High St., Suite C
		Longview, TX 75601, USA

5.3.2 *RCA Benefits and Drawbacks*

Today, RCA is widely used to investigate major industrial accidents. Some of its benefits are a well structured and process-focused approach, an effective tool to identify and address systems and organizational issues, and the systematic application of the method can uncover common root causes that link a disparate collection of accidents.[16]

In contrast some of the drawbacks associated with RCA are as follows[16]:

- It is a time-consuming and labor intensive approach.
- It is possible to be tainted by hindsight bias.
- In essence RCA is an uncontrolled case study.
- It is impossible to determine precisely, if the root cause established by the analysis is the actual cause of the accident.

5.4 Fault Tree Analysis (FTA)

This is a widely used method in the industry, particularly in nuclear power generation, to evaluate engineering systems during their design and development with respect to reliability and safety. A fault tree is a logical representation of the relationship of basic or primary events that may cause the occurrence of a given undesirable event, known as the "top event" and it is depicted using a tree structure with usually AND and OR logic gates.

The FTA approach was developed in the early 1960s at the Bell Telephone Laboratories to perform the analysis of the Minuteman Launch Control System with respect to reliability and safety. The method is described in detail in Ref. 9 and a comprehensive list of publications on the approach is given in Ref. 17.

5.4.1   *Fault Tree Symbols and Steps for Performing FTA*

There are many symbols used in the construction of fault trees. Figure 5.1 presents five such symbols obtained from Refs. 18 and 19. A circle denotes a basic fault event or the failure of an elementary component. The values of the event's parameters such as the occurrence probability, the occurrence/failure rate, and the repair rate are normally obtained from empirical data. A rectangle denotes a fault event that results from the logical combination of fault events through the input of a logic gate such as AND and OR. The diamond represents a fault event whose cause have not been fully developed due to factors such as the lack of required information or the lack of interest. The AND gate means that an output fault event occurs only if all the input fault events occur. The OR gate means that an output fault event occurs if any one or more input fault events should occur.

Usually, the following steps are used in performing the FTA[20]:

- Define the system and its associated assumptions.
- Identify the undesirable or the top fault event to be investigated (e.g. system failure).

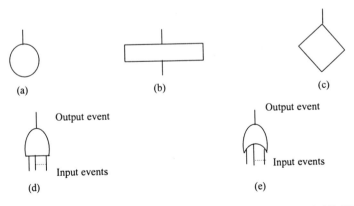

Fig. 5.1.   Basic fault tree symbols: (a) circle, (b) rectangle, (c) diamond, (d) AND gate, (e) OR gate.

- Determine all the possible causes that can lead to the occurrence of the top event by using fault tree symbols, such as those shown in Fig. 5.1, and the logic tree format.
- Develop the fault tree to the lowest level of detail as indicated by the requirements.
- Analyze the completed fault tree with respect to factors such as gaining insight into the unique modes of item/product faults and understanding the logic and the interrelationships among the various fault paths.
- Determine the most appropriate corrective actions.
- Document the analysis and follow up, as appropriate as possible, on the identified corrective actions.

Example 5.1 A hospitalized patient receives a medication from a nurse prescribed by a doctor. The patient can be given the wrong medication or an incorrect amount either due to nursing or doctor error. The nursing error can occur due to three causes: haste, poor work environment, and the incorrect interpretation of the doctor's instructions. Similarly, the doctor error can occur due to haste, poor surroundings, or misdiagnosis. Develop a fault tree for the top event "patient given wrong medication or incorrect amount" by using the symbols from Fig. 5.1.

A fault tree for the example is shown in Fig. 5.2. The single capital alphabet letters denote corresponding fault events (e.g. B: poor work environment, C: haste, and D: misdiagnosis).

5.4.2 *Probability Evaluation of Fault Trees*

When the probability of the occurrence of basic fault events is known, the probability of occurrence of the top event can easily be computed. This can only be obtained by first estimating the occurrence probability of the output fault events of the lower and intermediate logic gates such as the OR and the AND gates. The occurrence probability of the OR gate output fault event is given by[9]:

$$P(X_0) = 1 - \prod_{i=1}^{n} \{1 - P(X_i)\}, \tag{5.1}$$

where

$\quad P(X_0)$ is the OR gate output fault event, X_0, occurrence probability,
$\quad\quad n$ is the total number of input fault events, and

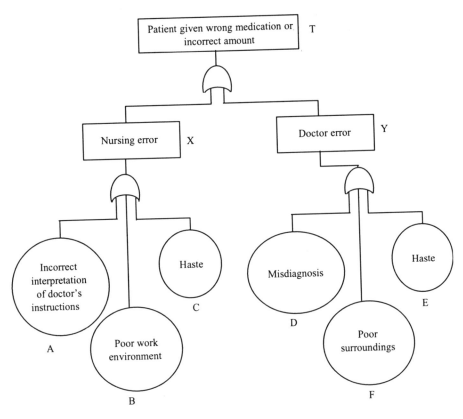

Fig. 5.2.   A fault tree for Example 5.1.

$P(X_i)$ is the probability of occurrence of OR gate input fault
event X_i; for $i = 1, 2, 3, \ldots, n$.

Similarly, the occurrence probability of the AND gate output fault event,
Y_0, is given by

$$P(Y_0) = \prod_{i=1}^{m} P(Y_i), \qquad (5.2)$$

where
   $P(Y_0)$ is the AND gate output fault event, Y_0, occurrence probability,
   m is the total number of input fault events, and
   $P(Y_i)$ is the probability of the occurrence of AND gate input fault
event Y_i; for $i = 1, 2, 3, \ldots, m$.

Example 5.2   Assume that the probabilities of occurrence of events A, B, C, D, E, and F in Fig. 5.2 are 0.01, 0.02, 0.03, 0.04, 0.05, and 0.06, respectively. Calculate the probability of occurrence of the top event T: patient given wrong medication or incorrect amount.

By substituting the occurrence probability values of the given events A, B, and C into Eq. 5.1, the probability of the nursing error, X, is:

$$P(X) = -1 - (1 - 0.01)(1 - 0.02)(1 - 0.03)$$
$$= 0.0589.$$

Similarly, by inserting the occurrence probability values of the specified events D, E, and F into Eq. 5.1, the probability of the doctor error, Y, is

$$P(Y) = -1 - (1 - 0.04)(1 - 0.05)(1 - 0.06)$$
$$= 0.1427.$$

Substituting the above two calculated values into Eq. 5.1, we get:

$$P(T) = -1 - (1 - 0.0589)(1 - 0.1427)$$
$$= 0.1932,$$

where $P(T)$ is the probability of occurrence of the top event.

Thus, the probability of the patient being given the wrong medication or incorrect amount is 0.1932. Figure 5.3 shows the fault tree from Fig. 5.2 with the above given and calculated fault event occurrence probability values.

5.5   Cause and Effect Diagram (CAED)

This method was developed in the early 1950s by K. Ishikawa, a Japanese quality expert. The method is also known as the Ishikawa diagram or the "Fishbone diagram" because of its resemblance to the skeleton of a fish. More specifically, the right hand side of the diagram (i.e. the fish head) represents the effect, and the left hand side displays all the possible causes which are linked to the central line called the "Fish Spine".

The cause and effect diagram could be very useful in determining the root causes of a given human error-related problem in health care. The main steps used in developing a CAED are as follows[20]:

- First, establish the problem statement.

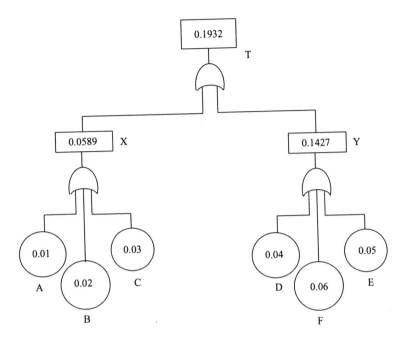

Fig. 5.3. A fault tree with fault event occurrence probability values.

- Brainstorm to identify all possible causes.
- Establish the major cause groups by stratifying them into natural categories and the steps of the process.
- Construct the diagram by connecting the identified causes under appropriate process steps and fill in the problem or the effect in the diagram box (i.e. the fish head) on the extreme right-hand side.
- Refine the cause categories by asking questions such as these listed below:

  — What causes this?
  — What is the reason for the existence of this condition?

Some of the advantages of the cause and effect diagram are shown in Fig. 5.4.

5.6   Hazard Operability Study (HAZOP)

This is an important method of safety analysis and it was originally developed in the chemical industry to perform safety-related studies.

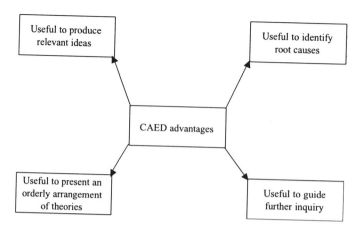

Fig. 5.4. Cause and effect diagram (CAED) advantages.

The method is quite useful in identifying problems before the complete data concerning an item is available. The method calls for the establishment of a team consisting of knowledgeable and experienced members with different backgrounds. In turn, the team members will brainstorm together about all possible potential hazards. The team is led by an experienced individual and during the brainstorming sessions, the same individual will act as a facilitator.

The main steps associated with HAZOP are as follows[21]:

- Select an item/product/system to be analyzed.
- Form a team of desirable and experienced individuals.
- Describe with care and in detail the HAZOP process to all the team members.
- Establish goals and appropriate time schedules.
- Conduct brainstorming sessions as deemed necessary.
- Document the final results.

One important disadvantage of the method is that it does not take into account the occurrence of human error in the final equation. The technique is described in detail in Ref. 22.

5.7 Probability Tree Method

This method is quite useful in performing task analysis by diagrammatically representing critical human actions and other related events. Often, this approach is used for conducting task analysis in the technique for the human error rate prediction (THERP).[23] Diagrammatic task analysis is denoted by the branches of the probability tree. More specifically, the branching limbs of the tree denote each event's outcome (i.e. success or failure) and each branch is assigned an occurrence probability.

There are many advantages of the probability tree method including simplified mathematical computations, itself being a visibility tool, and the flexibility to incorporate (i.e. with some modifications) factors such as emotional stress, interaction stress, and interaction effects. The method is described in detail in Ref. 23. The following example describes the basics of the probability tree method.

Example 5.3   Assume that a health care professional performs two tasks: "a" and "b". Task "a" is performed before task "b" and each task can either be performed correctly or incorrectly. Develop a probability tree and obtain an expression for the probability of not successfully accomplishing the overall mission. Assume that tasks "a" and "b" are performed independently. More specifically, the performance of task "a" does not affect the performance of task "b" or vice-versa.

In this case, the health care professional first performs task "a" correctly or incorrectly and then proceeds to perform task "b". Task "b" can also be performed correctly or incorrectly. A probability tree shown in Fig. 5.5 depicts this scenario.

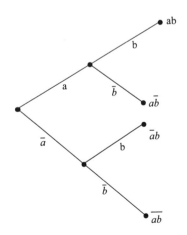

Fig. 5.5.   Probability tree for performing tasks "a" and "b".

The symbols used in the figure are defined below:

a   denotes the event that task "a" is performed successfully,
b   denotes the event that task "b" is performed successfully,
$\bar{a}$ denotes the event that task "a" is performed incorrectly, and
$\bar{b}$ denotes the event that task "b" is performed incorrectly.

In Fig. 5.5 "ab" denote the overall mission success. Thus, the probability of occurrence of events "ab" is

$$P(ab) = P_a P_b, \tag{5.3}$$

where

P_a is the probability of performing task "a" correctly, and
P_b is the probability of performing task "b" correctly.

Similarly, in Fig. 5.5 $a\bar{b}$, $\bar{a}b$, and $\overline{ab}$ denote the three distinct possibilities of having an overall mission failure. Thus, the probability of not successfully accomplishing the overall mission is

$$P_f = P(a\bar{b} + \bar{a}b + \overline{ab}) = P_a P_{\bar{b}} + P_{\bar{a}} P_b + P_{\bar{a}} P_{\bar{b}}, \tag{5.4}$$

where

$P_{\bar{a}}$ is the probability of performing task "a" incorrectly,
$P_{\bar{b}}$ is the probability of performing task "b" incorrectly, and
P_f is the probability of not successfully accomplishing the overall mission.

Example 5.4   Assume that in Example 5.3, the probabilities of the health care professional performing tasks "a" and "b" correctly are 0.8 and 0.9, respectively. Calculate the probabilities of successfully and unsuccessfully accomplishing the overall mission by the professional.

By substituting the given values into Eq. 5.3, we get:

$$P(ab) = (0.8)(0.9) = 0.72.$$

Since $P_a + P_{\bar{a}} = 1$ and $P_b + P_{\bar{b}} = 1$, by inserting the specified values into Eq. 5.4, we get:

$$P_f = (0.8)(1 - 0.9) + (1 - 0.8)(0.9) + (1 - 0.8)(1 - 0.9)$$
$$= 0.08 + 0.18 + 0.02$$
$$= 0.28.$$

The probabilities of successfully and unsuccessfully accomplishing the overall mission by the health care professional are 0.72 and 0.28, respectively.

5.8   Error-Cause Removal Program (ECRP)

This method was developed to reduce human error to some tolerable level in production operations.[24] Its emphasis is on preventive measures rather than merely on remedial ones. ECRP may simply be called the production worker-participation program for reducing the occurrence of human errors. Some examples of production workers are: assembly personnel, inspection personnel, machinists, and maintenance workers. More specifically, the ECRP is made up of teams of production workers with each team having its own coordinator. The coordinator possesses special technical and group related skills and the maximum size of the team is twelve persons. Team meetings are held periodically, in which the workers present their error and error-likely reports. The reports are discussed and recommendations are made for remedial or preventive measures. These recommendations are presented to the management by the team coordinators for action to be taken.

Human factors specialist and other specialists then assist both management and the team with regards to factors such as evaluations and implementations of the suggested design solutions. Three important guidelines associated with the ECRP are as follows:

- Carefully evaluate each work redesign recommended by the team with regards to factors such as the degree of error reduction, the increment in job satisfaction and cost-effectiveness.
- Restrict to the identification of work conditions that require redesign for reducing the occurrence of error potential.
- Focus on data collection in errors, accident-prone conditions, and error-likely situations.

All in all, ECRP comprises of the following seven basic components[25]:

- Each and every individual associated with the ECRP is properly educated about its usefulness.
- The production workers' efforts with respect to ECRP are recognized by the management in an appropriate manner.
- The most promising proposed design solutions are implemented by the management.

- All team coordinators and workers are trained in data collection and analysis methods.
- Human factors and other specialists evaluate the effects of changes in the production process with the aid of the ECRP inputs.
- Production workers report and determine errors and error-likely conditions. Furthermore, the workers propose design solutions to eradicate error causes.
- The proposed design solutions are evaluated with respect to cost by human factors and other specialists.

5.9   Man-Machine Systems Analysis (MMSA)

This method was developed in the early 1950s to reduce human-error-caused unwanted effects to some acceptable level in a given system.[26] The method comprises of the following ten steps[26]:

- Define the system functions and goals.
- Define the situational characteristics. More specifically, the performance-shaping factors such as illumination, quality of air, and union actions under which humans have to perform their tasks.
- Define the characteristics of the persons involved. Some examples of these characteristics are experience, training, motivation, and skills.
- Define the tasks/jobs performed by the manpower involved.
- Conduct with care the analysis of tasks/jobs for the purpose of highlighting potential error-likely situations and other related difficulties.
- Estimate the chances or other information with respect to the occurrence of each potential human error.
- Estimate the likelihood that each potential human error will remain undetected and unrectified.
- Determine the consequences if potential errors are undetected.
- Make appropriate recommendations for changes.
- Re-evaluate each change by repeating most of the above steps.

All in all, with some modifications this method can also be used in the health care system.

5.10   Markov Method

This is a powerful method often used in reliability and safety studies and it can probably cover more cases than any other method in these areas. The method is known after a Russian mathematician named Andrei Andreyevich Markov (1856–1922).

The method is quite useful in modeling operation systems with dependent failure and repair modes. In fact, it is widely used to perform reliability and availability analyses of repairable systems with constant failure and repair rates. From time to time, the Markov method is also used to perform human reliability analysis.[25]

The following assumptions are associated with this approach[26]:

- The probability of the occurrence of a transition from one system state to another in the finite time interval Δt is given by $\theta \Delta t$, where θ is the transition rate from one system state to another.
- The transition probability of more than one occurrences in time interval Δt from one state to another is negligible (e.g. $(\theta \Delta t)(\theta \Delta t) \to 0$).
- All occurrences are independent of each other.

The following example demonstrates the application of the Markov method in the health care human reliability analysis.

Example 5.5 A health care professional performs his or her tasks in normal environment and makes errors at a constant rate θ. More specifically, a state space diagram describing this scenario is shown in Fig. 5.6. Develop expressions for the health care professional's reliability and unreliability at time t by using the Markov method.

Using the Markov method, we write down the following equations for Fig. 5.6:

$$P_0(t + \Delta t) = P_0(t)(1 - \theta \Delta t), \tag{5.5}$$

$$P_1(t + \Delta t) = P_1(t) + P_0(t)\theta \Delta t, \tag{5.6}$$

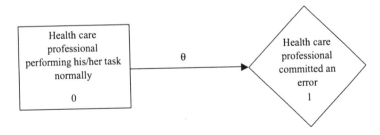

Fig. 5.6. State space diagram representing the health care professional. The numerals in the figure denote system states.

where

t is time,

$P_0(t)$ is the probability that the health care professional is performing his/her task normally (i.e. state 0 in Fig. 5.6) at time t,

$P_1(t)$ is the probability that the health care professional has committed an error (i.e. state 1 in Fig. 5.6) at time t,

θ is the constant error rate of the health care professional,

$\theta \Delta t$ is the probability of human error by the health care professional in finite time interval Δt,

$(1 - \theta \Delta t)$ is the probability of zero human error by the health care professional in finite time interval Δt,

$P_0(t + \Delta t)$ is the probability that the health care professional is performing his/her task normally (i.e. state 0 in Fig. 5.6) at time $(t + \Delta t)$, and

$P_1(t + \Delta t)$ is the probability that the health care professional has committed an error (i.e. State 1 in Fig. 5.6) at time $(t + \Delta t)$.

By rearranging Eqs. 5.5–5.6, we write:

$$\lim_{\Delta t \to 0} \frac{P_0(t + \Delta t) - P_0(t)}{\Delta t} = -\theta P_0(t), \tag{5.7}$$

$$\lim_{\Delta t \to 0} \frac{P_1(t + \Delta t) - P_1(t)}{\Delta t} = \theta P_0(t). \tag{5.8}$$

Thus, from Eqs. 5.7 and 5.8, we get:

$$\frac{dP_0(t)}{dt} + \theta P_0(t) = 0, \tag{5.9}$$

$$\frac{dP_1(t)}{dt} - \theta P_0(t) = 0. \tag{5.10}$$

At time $t = 0$, $P_0(0) = 1$ and $P_1(0) = 0$.

Solving Eqs. 5.9–5.10 by using Laplace transforms, we get:

$$P_0(s) = \frac{1}{s + \theta}, \tag{5.11}$$

$$P_1(s) = \frac{\theta}{s(s + \theta)}, \tag{5.12}$$

where s is the Laplace transform variable.

By taking the inverse Laplace transforms of Eqs. 5.11 and 5.12 yields

$$P_0(t) = e^{-\theta t}, \tag{5.13}$$
$$P_1(t) = 1 - e^{-\theta t}. \tag{5.14}$$

Expressions for the health care professional's reliability and unreliability at time t are given by Eqs. 5.13 and 5.14, respectively.

Example 5.6   Assume that the error rate of a health care professional performing a certain task is 0.007 errors/hour. Calculate the reliability and unreliability of the health care professional during a 10-hour work period.

Using the given values in Eqs. 5.13 and 5.14, we get:

$$P_0(10) = e^{-(0.007)(10)}$$
$$= 0.9324, \text{ and}$$
$$P_1(10) = 1 - e^{-(0.007)(10)}$$
$$= 0.0676.$$

Thus, the health care professional's reliability and unreliability are 0.9324 and 0.0676, respectively.

Problems

1. Write an essay on the history of failure modes and effect analysis (FMEA).
2. What is the difference between FMEA and failure mode effects and criticality analysis (FMECA)?
3. List at least eight important advantages of FMEA.
4. Discuss about the root cause analysis (RCA).
5. What are the important benefits and drawbacks of the RCA approach?
6. Describe the following terms with respect to fault tree analysis (FTA):

   - AND gate
   - OR gate
   - Top event
   - Basic fault event

7. Compare FTA with FMEA.
8. Describe the following two methods:

   - Cause and effect diagram (CAED).
   - Hazard and operability study (HAZOP).

9. Make a comparison between FMEA and HAZOP.
10. A nurse is performing a certain task and her hourly error rate is 0.0002 errors. Compute the nurse's unreliability during an 7-hour mission.

References

1. Omdahl, T.P., (ed), *Reliability, Availability, and Maintainability (RAM) Dictionary*, American Society for Quality Control (ASQC) Press, Milwaukee, Wisconsin, 1988.
2. Mil-F-18372 (Aer.), *General Specification for Design, Installation, and Test of Aircraft Flight Control Systems*, Bureau of Naval Weapons, Department of the Navy, Washington, D.C., Paragraph 3.5.2.3.
3. Continho, J.S., "Failure Effect Analysis," *Transactions of the New York Academy of Sciences*, Vol. 26, Series II, 1963–1964, pp. 564–584.
4. Jordan, W.E., "Failure Modes, Effects and Criticality Analyses," *Proceedings of the Annual Reliability and Maintainability Symposium*, 1972, pp. 30–37.
5. MIL-STD-1629, *Procedures for Performing a Failure Mode, Effects, and Criticality Analysis*, Department of Defense, Washington, D.C., 1980.
6. Dhillon, B.S., "Failure Mode and Effects Analysis: Bibliography," *Microelectronics and Reliability*, Vol. 32, 1992, pp. 719–731.
7. Dhillon, B.S., *Systems Reliability, Maintainability, and Management*, Petrocelli Book, Inc., New York, 1983.
8. Palady, P., *Failure Modes and Effects Analysis*, PT Publications, West Palm Beach, Florida, 1995.
9. Dhillon, B.S., *Design Reliability: Fundamentals and Applications*, CRC Press, Inc., Boca Raton, Florida, 1999.
10. Busse, D.K. and Wright, D.J., *Classification and Analysis of Incidents in Complex, Medical Environments*, Report, 2000, Available from the Intensive Care Unit, Western General Hospital, Edinburgh, UK.
11. Latino, R.J., *Automating Root Cause Analysis, in Error Reduction in Health Care*, edited by P.L. Spath, John Wiley and Sons, New York, 2000, pp. 155–164.
12. Feldman, S.E. and Roblin, D.W., "Accident Investigation and Anticipatory Failure Analysis in Hospitals," in *Error Reduction in Health Care*, edited by P. L. Spath, John Wiley and Sons, New York, 2000, pp. 139–154.
13. Lement, B.S. and Ferrera, J.J., "Accident Causation Analysis by Technical Experts," *Journal of Product Liability*, Vol. 5, No. 2, 1982, pp. 145–160.
14. Hirsch, K.A. and Wallace, D.T., *Conducting Root Cause Analysis in a Health Care Environment*, Report, 2001, Available from the Medical Risk Management Associates, San Diego, California.
15. Burke, A., *Root Cause Analysis*, Report, 2002, Available from the Wild Iris Medical Education, P.O. Box 257, Comptche, California.
16. Wald, H. and Shojania, K.G., "Root Cause Analysis," in *Making Health Care Safer: A Critical Analysis of Patient Safety Practices*, edited by A.J.

Markowitz, Report No. 43, Agency for Health Care Research and Quality, US Department of Health and Human Services, Rockville, Maryland, 2001, Chapter 5, pp. 1–7.

17. Dhillon, B.S., *Reliability and Quality Control: Bibliography on General and Specialized Areas*, Beta Publishers, Inc., Gloucester, Ontario, Canada, 1992.

18. Schroder, R.J., "Fault Tree for Reliability Analysis," *Proceedings of the Annual Symposium on Reliability*, 1970, pp. 170–174.

19. Dhillon, B.S. and Singh, C., *Engineering Reliability: New Techniques and Applications*, John Wiley and Sons, New York, 1981.

20. Mears, P., *Quality Improvement Tools and Techniques*, McGraw Hill, Inc., New York, 1995.

21. *Risk Analysis Requirements and Guidelines*, Report No. CAN/CSA-Q634-91, prepared by the Canadian Standards Association, 1991, Available from Canadian Standards Association, 178 Rexdale Boulevard, Rexdale, Ontario, Canada.

22. Goetsch, D.L., *Occupational Safety and Health*, Prentice Hall, Inc., Englewood Cliffs, New Jersey, 1996.

23. Swain, A.D., *A Method for Performing a Human-factors Reliability Analysis*, Report No. SCR-685, Sandia Corporation, Albuquerque, New Mexico, August 1963.

24. Swain, A.D., "An Error-cause Removal Program for Industry," *Human Factors*, Vol. 12, 1973, pp. 207–221.

25. Dhillon, B.S., *Human Reliability: with Human Factors*, Pergamon Press, Inc., New York, 1986.

26. Miller, R.B., *A Method for Man-machine Task Analysis*, Report No. 53–137, Wright Air Development Center, Wright-Patterson Air Force Base, US Air Force (USAF), Ohio, 1953.

Chapter 6

Human Error in Medication

6.1 Introduction

Each day millions of people fall ill, and with the aid of modern medicine a vast number of them recover and they lead a healthy lifestyle thereafter. The process of prescribing and taking medicine is not one hundred percent reliable. More specifically, it is subjected to error because the individuals involved such as the nurses, pharmacists, doctors, or even the patients themselves make mistakes. Although medication errors are considered unacceptable, they probably occur more frequently than they are actually reported due to various factors including the loss of business or employment, the existence of poor or no error reporting systems at all, and the loss of personal or organizational prestige.

By examining various studies performed over the years, it can be established that medication errors are frequent and that adverse drug events or injuries due to drugs occur more frequently than what was deemed appropriate.[1-5] It may be said relatively that medication errors leading to death or serious injuries occur infrequently, but a sizable and an increasing number of individuals each year are affected because of the widespread use of drugs both within and outside the hospital environments.[6]

A medication error may simply be defined as any preventable event that may cause or result in wrong medication use or patient harm while the medication is in the control of a patient, a consumer, or a health-care professional.[7] This chapter presents various different aspects of human error in medication.

6.2   Medication Error Facts, Figures, and Examples

Some of the facts and examples that are directly or indirectly concerned with medication errors are as follows:

- In 1993, 7391 people died due to medication errors in the United States.[6,8]
- In 1998, approximately 2.5 billion prescriptions were dispensed in pharmacies, in the United States, at an estimated cost of around $92 billion.[6,9]
- The cost of medication errors is estimated to be over $7 billion per year in the United States.[10]
- The annual cost of hospital-based medication related errors is estimated to be around $2 billion in the United States.[11]
- In 1993, over a ten-year period outpatient deaths due to medication errors increased by 8.48-fold in the United States as opposed to a 2.37-fold increase in inpatient deaths.[6,8]
- A university professor of pharmacy believes that around 200000 Americans die due to medication mistakes each year.[12]
- An examination of fourteen Australian studies published during the period from 1988 to 1996 revealed that 2.4 to 3.6% of all hospital admissions were drug related and around 32 to 69% were preventable.[6,13]
- In 1986, a review of seven studies, conducted in the United States, revealed that 5.5% of hospital admissions, i.e. 1.94 million admissions, can be attributed to drug therapy noncompliance. Their total cost to hospitals was estimated to be around $8.5 billion.[6,14]
- In 2000, around 50% of the chain pharmacy store executives in the United States responding to a survey indicated that they had instituted new measures to prevent or reduce prescribed drug errors in response to the startling findings, concerning medical errors, in the Institute of Medicine (IOM) report released in 1999.[6,15]
- In 1991, a 77 year old woman was inadvertently given 250 mg of acetohexamide (Dymelor), an oral hypoglycemic, instead of 250 mg of acetazolamide (Diamox) for glaucoma.[16]
- A 30 year old woman with asthma experienced palpitation and visited her regular general practitioner. In turn, the practitioner erroneously prescribed a Badrenoceptor antagonist. After taking the first tablet of the prescribed drug, the woman collapsed and died later.[17,18]
- Medication errors range from 5.3% to 20.6% of administered doses.[19]
- At one time the antidote for paracetamol poisoning, N-acetylcysteine, was administered at ten times the right amount to twenty patients and two of them died later.[20]

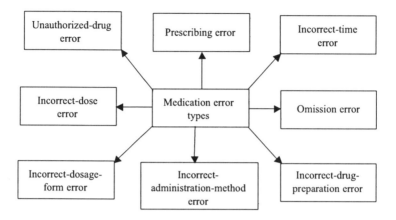

Fig. 6.1.   Types of medication errors.

6.3   Types and Causes of Medication Error and Medication Use Processes

There are basically eight types of medication errors as shown in Fig. 6.1.[7,21] Omission error is simply the oversight in administering a recommended dose to a patient prior to the next scheduled dose (if any). Unauthorized-drug error is the administration of medication not recommended by the patient's legitimate prescriber. Incorrect-administration-method error is the wrong procedure or the wrong method used in the administration of a drug. Incorrect-drug-preparation error occurs when the drug product is wrongly formulated or is manipulated prior to administration.

Prescribing error is the wrong drug selection, quantity, rate of administration, dose, dosage form, concentration, route, or instructions for use of a drug product authorized by the legitimate prescriber. Furthermore, prescribing error can also be illegible prescriptions or medication orders that result in errors suffered by the patient. Some typical examples of prescribing errors are presented in Table 6.1.[22]

Incorrect-dosage-form error is the administration of a drug product to the patient in varying dosage other than the dosage recommended by the legitimate prescriber. Incorrect-time error is the administration of medication outside a predefined time interval from its already scheduled administration time. Finally, incorrect-dose error is the administration to the patient a dose that is higher than or lower than the amount recommended by the legitimate prescriber.

Table 6.1.   Typical examples of prescribing errors.

No.	Error Example
1	A physician prescribed Septra to a patient allergic to sulfa.
2	Dosage unadjusted for age, body size, or renal insufficiency.
3	Medication mistimed with respect to bedtime or meals.
4	A physician prescribed erythromycin to a patient already on theophylline.
5	A physician prescribed aspirin to a patient with asthma.
6	Failure to obtain indicated chemistry or hematology values to monitor for potential toxicities.

Although, there are many causes for the occurrence of medication errors, some of the common ones are as follows[7]:

- Illegible handwriting
- Designation of ambiguous strength on labels or in packaging
- Wrong dosage calculation
- Errors in labeling
- Equipment malfunction
- Wrong transcription
- Drug product nomenclature (e.g. use of numbered or lettered suffixes and prefixes in drug names)
- Medication is not available
- Poorly trained personnel
- Excessive workload
- Incorrect abbreviations used during the prescribing process
- Lapses in individual performance

Ensuring proper medication use is a very complex process. It involves multiple organizations and individuals from different disciplines, timely access to complete and correct patient related information, a series of inter-related decisions over a time period, and the mastering of a proper knowledge of the drug. Nonetheless, major elements of medication use processes are shown in Fig. 6.2.[6] These elements are subjected to the occurrence of commission and omission errors. Two typical examples of commission and omission errors are the administration of improper drug and the failure to administer a prescribed drug, respectively. Nonetheless, Fig. 6.2 shows five major elements of medication use processes, namely: prescribing, dispensing, administering, monitoring, as well as systems and management

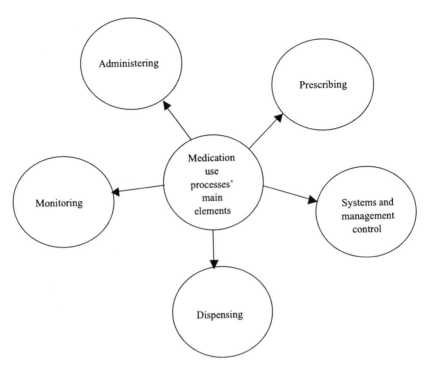

Fig. 6.2.   Major elements of medication use processes.

control. Various tasks (in parentheses) are associated with each of these elements: prescribing (i.e. determining the need for a drug, choosing the correct drug, designating the desired therapeutic response, and individualizing the therapeutic regimen), dispensing (i.e. reviewing and processing the order, dispensing the drug on time, and compounding and preparing the drug), administering (i.e. administering the appropriate medication to the right patient, administering medication as indicated, informing the patient about the medication, and including the patient in administration), monitoring (i.e. monitoring and documenting the patient's response, re-evaluating drug selection, regimen, frequency, and time duration, as well as identifying and reporting adverse drug events), and systems and management control (i.e. reviewing and managing the patient's complete therapeutic drug regimen, as well as collaborating and communicating amongst caregivers).

6.4   Medication Errors in Hospitals, Nursing Factors in Medication Errors, and Medication Errors Leading to Manslaughter Charges

Medication errors occur quite frequently in hospitals. Two examples of the findings concerned with medication errors in hospitals are as follows[6]:

- A review of 289411 medication orders written during a 12-month period in a tertiary-care teaching hospital reported that the overall error rate was 3.13 errors per 1000 orders written and the rate of significant errors was around 1.81 per 1000 orders.
- A review of 36653 hospitalized patients identified 731 adverse drug events (ADEs) in 648 patients, out of which only 92 were reported by nurses, physicians, and pharmacists and the remaining ADEs were discovered through other means.

Additional studies, that may directly or indirectly relate to medication errors in hospitals, are presented in a subsequent section of this chapter.

Past experiences indicate that a significant proportion of medication errors can be attributed to nurses. In turn, there are many factors that play an instrumental role in the occurrence of nursing-related medication errors. Some of these are as follows[23]:

- **Nurses' knowledge of medication.** As the nurses are accountable for the drug they administer, they must possess a good knowledge of the action, side-effects (if any), and the right dosage of any drugs they handle. Over the years, the need for the nurses to continuously update their knowledge of drugs have increased greatly with the increasing number of drugs available for administration in hospitals and in the community.[24] Past experiences indicate that the lack of knowledge appears to be a persistent problem in the occurrence of medication errors. For example, as indicated in Ref. 25 29% of the 334 medication errors investigated were due to the lack of drug knowledge among the nurses, doctors, and the pharmacists.
- **Nurses' mathematical skills.** Proficiency in mathematical skills is absolutely necessary in performing various nursing functions including intravenous regulations, medication calculations, as well as intake and output calculations.[26] Past experiences indicate that many medication errors have resulted because of the poor mathematical skills of the nurses.[26,27]

- **Length of nursing experience.** Presently research in relation to nursing experience and medication errors appears to be inconclusive. Nonetheless, it may be said that nurses new to the hospitals are more likely to make mistakes, probably due to the new environment. At the same time, it may be added that these nurses are also more likely to report errors than those employed for longer periods.[23]

- **Nursing shifts.** A number of researchers have concluded that a variety of working conditions, including shift rotation, contribute to the occurrence of medication errors.[23,28–29] For example, Refs. 23 and 28 state that more nursing related medication errors occur during the day shift than during the evening or night-time shifts, and nurses who work through different shifts are twice as likely to make errors, respectively.

- **Nurses' workload and staffing level.** Past data have indicated that the amount of workload carried by the nurses also affect the rate of occurrence of medication errors.[23,25,30] Also, as the shortage of nursing manpower increases the number of medication administrations per nurse. In a way this may increase the probability of the occurrence of medication errors.[31]

- **Drug administration.** Although some researchers believe that a single-nurse drug administration does not increase the number of errors,[23,32] but as indicated by Ref. 33, two-nurse drug administration generates fewer mistakes as compared to the single-nurse drug administration.

- **Adherence to policy and procedures.** Although medication administration polices and procedures exist in hospitals and other facilities, the failure to adhere to such policies and procedures is an on-going problem.[23,30] This is a potential source of medication errors generated by the nurses. Nonetheless, as indicated by Ref. 34 around 72% of the medication errors can be attributable to the failure of staff members in following policies and procedures.

- **Written prescription quality.** Often nurses come across poorly written and even illegible prescriptions. This generates a potential for medication errors. For example, as stated in Ref. 35 nurses often administer medications in an unsafe manner due to poorly written prescriptions.

- **Distractions and interruptions.** From time to time distractions and interruptions are cited as a factor in the occurrence of medication errors by the nurses.[23,36] Moreover, a survey of 175 nurses reported that 32% of them consider frequent interruptions or distractions as factors contributing to medication error.[30]

Doctors and other health care professionals are expected to exercise proper care in their daily work activities. In the event of their negligence, when harm is done to the patients, these professionals may face increasing criticisms or even civil actions from their patients. For example, there were a total of seventeen charges brought against twenty-one doctors, accusing them of manslaughter due to errors in drug treatment/anesthesia for the period of 1970–1999 in the United Kingdom alone.[17] Two cases of these manslaughter charges are briefly discussed below[17]:

- A 41 year old woman with severe migraine was given prochlorperazine and diazepam by a general practitioner. Subsequent to its failure in relieving her pain, the same practitioner administered her an ampoule containing 100 mg of diamorphine. The woman died within an hour and the practitioner was charged with manslaughter.
- A state enrolled nurse administered 300 mg of morphine to a wrong patient in a nursing home. Subsequently, a general practitioner simply recommended careful observations of the patient. The patient collapsed and died later. All nurses involved and the general practitioner were charged with manslaughter.

6.5   Medication Error Reduction

The occurrence of medication errors has become a pressing issue and various measures have been proposed to reduce their occurrence. Some of these measures are presented below.

6.5.1   *Use of Information Technology for Reducing Medication Errors in Hospitals*

In the past, several interventions involving information systems/technology have been shown to reduce the occurrence of medication errors. For example, as stated in Ref. 12 the usage of a computerized drug-ordering system has reduced medication error-related deaths in one hospital by 55%. The following information technology-related items are useful in reducing medication errors in hospitals[5]:

- **Computerized physician order entry (CPOE).** This may simply be described as an application in which physicians write orders online.

CPOE helps to improve safety in several ways including having structured orders (they include a dose, route, and frequency), being legible and having the ability to identify the physician and the prescriptions at all instances, being able to check all orders for various problems (e.g. allergies, drug interactions, and overly high doses), and being able to provide information to the physician during the process. Past experiences indicate that the use of COPE has helped to reduce medication errors dramatically, e.g. in one case by 64% and in another by 83%.[37]

- **Computerized adverse drug event detection.** In order to monitor the effectiveness of any process, it is absolutely necessary to have the ability to measure its outcomes. Nonetheless, computerized data are useful in detecting signals (e.g. a high concentration of a drug or the use of an antidote) that are related to an adverse reaction.[38,39] All in all, it may be said that computerized monitoring is probably the first practical approach in monitoring the medication process on a continuous basis and its cost is around 20% of the chart review approach cost.

- **Automated medication administration records.** The medication administration record system is used by clinicians to keep records of prescribed drugs. The computerization of this system, particularly when linked to the computerized physician order entry system, could be quite useful in reducing the occurrence of medication errors.

- **Use of robots for filling prescriptions.** Although robots are being used in the outpatient setting in some hospitals, their use in filling prescriptions could help to reduce medication errors. As stated in Ref. 5 the use of a robot in the dispensing area has resulted in a reduction in the dispensing error rate from 2.9% to 0.6%.

- **Bar coding.** Although bar coding is widely used in many industries outside the medical field, it can be useful for immediate assurance that the drug at hand is actually the intended one. It can also be used to identify and record personnels giving and receiving the drug. In some hospitals in the United States, bar coding is already being used. In particular, one hospital has already reported an 80% reduction in medication administration errors with the use of bar coding.[5]

- **Automated dispensing devices.** These devices can be employed to withhold the drugs at a specified location and to dispense them only to a specified patient. The occurrence of medication errors decreases substantially when these devices are linked with bar coding and are interfaced with the hospital information systems.[40,41]

6.5.2   *Role of Manufacturers and Food and Drug Administration (FDA) in Reducing Medication Errors*

Increased attention on medication safety has applied pressure on manufacturers to carefully examine the industrial procedures to reduce the occurrence of medication errors. The Institute of Medicine (IOM) report entitled "To Err is Human: Building a Safer Health Care System" recommends the FDA to take action in the following three areas[10]:

- **Drug packaging and labeling.** In this area, the report calls for the FDA to develop and enforce standards for the design of drug packaging and labeling that will maximize safety in product usage throughout the United States. Furthermore, IOM wants the FDA to extend its medical device program (that encourages manufacturers to extend human factors analysis with respect to product misuse) to drugs as well.
- **Drug-name confusion.** In this area, the IOM report suggests that the FDA should require pharmaceutical companies to look into proposed drug names to prevent sound-alike confusions, thus reducing medication errors.
- **Post-marketing surveillance.** In this area, the IOM report suggests that the FDA should perform both intensive and extensive monitoring to highlight problems immediately after a newly manufactured product appears on the market and it should also take immediate actions should serious risks to public health arise. These steps should help to reduce medication errors directly or indirectly.

6.5.3   *General Guidelines for Reducing Medication Errors*

Over the years various general guidelines have been developed for medical professionals to reduce medication-related errors. Some of these guidelines are as follows[7,22]:

- Pay careful attention to safety and efficacy when determining the amount of drug to be prescribed.
- Write legibly or make use of computer-generated prescriptions.
- Provide clear and concise verbal and written medication instructions.
- Verbally educate patients on the name and purpose of each medication.
- Avoid distractions during the preparation of medication for administration.

- Enquire from the patient about his/her allergies prior to administering any medication.
- Avoid leaving medications by the patient's bedside.
- Perform calculations of dosages on paper, not in the head.
- Seriously consider the possibility of inadvertent drug substitutions when some side effects are reported by the patient.
- Gain some knowledge of the patient's diagnosis to ensure the correctness of the drug.
- Check the drug label three times (i.e. at the time of removing the container from storage, prior to administering the drug and before discarding or returning the container).
- Check the identification bracelet of each patient prior to administering a medication.
- Check the chart for allergies with care when checking the medication administration record (MAR) against the doctor's orders.
- Ensure that the patient's allergy alert is on the MAR and the front of the chart.
- Review the original order with care against the patient's MAR well within 24-hours to check for any transcription errors.

6.6 Medication Error-Related Studies

Over the years many studies directly or indirectly concerned with medication errors have been performed. Some of these studies are presented below[6]:

- **Knox Study.**[42] This study was concerned with the analysis of medication errors made by 51 Massachusetts pharmacists. The study found that 88% of medication errors involved incorrect drug or incorrect dose and 63% involved first-time prescriptions rather than refills. Pharmacists cited various factors for the occurrence of errors: too many telephone calls (62% of the pharmacists), unusually busy day (59% of the pharmacists), too many customers (53% of the pharmacists), lack of concentration (41% of the pharmacists), and staff shortage (32% of the pharmacists).
- **Nolan and O'Malley Study.**[6] This study reports the result of 21 hospital inpatient studies performed in the Untied States, New Zealand, Israel, United Kingdom, and Switzerland. According to the study, even though the percentage of patients experiencing ADRs ranged from 1.5%

to 43.5%, the majority of the remaining studies documented ADR rates between 10% and 25%.

- **Wilson *et al. Study*.**[43] This study was concerned with 682 children admitted to a Congential Heart Disease Center at a teaching hospital in the United Kingdom. The study found a total of 441 medical errors in three areas: prescription (68%), administration (25%), and supply (7%). The breakdown of these errors among the medical professionals were: doctors (72%), nurses (22%), pharmacy staff (5%), and doctors/nurses combination (1%).

- **Bates *et al. Study*.**[44] This study was concerned with a cohart of 379 consecutive admissions during a 51-day period in three medical units of an urban tertiary care hospital. The study found that out of the 10070 medication orders written, a total of 530 medication errors were made (i.e. 5.3 errors per 100 orders). Five of the 530 errors led to ADEs.

- **Leape *et al. Study*.**[25] This study was concerned with all non-obstetric adult admissions to eleven medical and surgical units in two tertiary care hospitals during the period between February and July 1993. The study reported a total of 334 errors as the causes of 264 potential and preventable ADEs. The causes of the errors were sixteen major system failures. Seven of these system failures accounted for 78% of the errors.

- **Brennan *et al. Study*.**[4] This study was concerned with 30195 randomly selected records in 51 hospitals in New York State in 1984 and out of which a total of 30121 records were actually reviewed by physicians. The study revealed the occurrence of ADEs in only 3.7% of hospitalizations. However, 70.5% of the ADEs gave rise to disabilities lasting less than six months, 13.6% resulted in deaths, and 2.6% caused permanent disabling injuries.

- **Lesar *et al. Study*.**[45] This study was concerned with 289411 medication orders written during the period from January 1, 1987 to December 31, 1987 in a tertiary care teaching hospital. The study discovered a total of 905 prescribing errors, out of which around 58% had a potential for adverse consequences. Furthermore, the study found the overall error rate of 3.13 per 1000 orders written along with the rate of significant errors of 1.81 per 1000 orders written.

- **Lazarou *et al. Study*.**[6] This study was concerned with 39 prospective studies from US hospitals in which four electronic databases were searched for incidents of adverse drug reactions in hospitalized patients between 1966 and 1996. The study found that out of the total incidents 6.7% were serious adverse drug reactions (ADRs) and 0.32% were fatal ADRs in hospitalized patients.

- **Bates *et al.* Study.**[6] This study was concerned with all patients admitted to two medical, two surgical, two obstetric general care units and one coronary intensive care unit over a period of 37 days in an urban tertiary care hospital. The study revealed the occurrence of 73 drug-related incidents in 2967 patient days, out of which 27 incidents were judged as ADEs, 34 were potential ADEs, and 12 were problem orders. Furthermore, 15 of the 27 ADEs were considered preventable. Moreover, 72% of the incidents were judged to be caused by physicians.

- **Folli *et al.* Study.**[46] This study was concerned with 101022 medication orders prescribed in two children's teaching hospitals over a period from February 1985 to July 1985. The study revealed a combined total of 479 errant medication orders. The most common and prevalent errors were wrong dosage and overdosage, respectively.

Problems

1. Define the term "medication error".
2. List at least five medication error-related facts and figures.
3. What are the types of medication errors?
4. Discuss at least ten common causes for the occurrence of medication errors.
5. Write down at least five typical examples of prescribing errors.
6. What are the major components of medication use processes?
7. What are the important nursing-related factors in the occurrence of medication errors?
8. Discuss at least two examples of manslaughter charges due to medication errors.
9. Discuss the use of information technology for reducing medication errors in hospitals.
10. List at least ten general guidelines for reducing the occurrence of medication errors.

References

1. Leape, L.L., Brennan, T.A., and Laird, N.M., *et al.*, "The Nature of Adverse Events in Hospitalized Patients: Results from the Harvard Medical Practice Study, II," *N. Eng. J. Med.*, Vol. 324, 1991, pp. 377–384.
2. Lazar, J., Pomeranz, B.H., and Corey, P.N., "Incidence of Adverse Drug Reactions in Hospitalized Patients: A Meta-analysis of Prospective Studies," *JAMA*, Vol. 279, 1998, pp. 1200–1205.

3. Bates, D.W., Cullen, D., Laird, N., *et al.*, "Incidence of Adverse Drug Events and Potential Adverse Drug Events: Implications for Prevention," *JAMA*, Vol. 274, 1995, pp. 29–34.

4. Brennan, T.A., Leepe, L.L., Laired, N., *et al.*, "Incidence of Adverse Events and Negligence in Hospitalized Patients: Results from Harvard Medical Practice Study I," *New England Journal Medicine*, Vol. 324, 1991, pp. 370–376.

5. Bates, D.W., "Using Information Technology to Reduce Rates of Medication Errors in Hospitals," *British Medical Journal*, Vol. 320, 2000, pp. 788–791.

6. Kohn, L., Corrigan, J., and Donaldson, M., (eds), *To Err is Human: Building a Safer Health System*, National Academy Press, Washington, D.C., 1999.

7. Coleman, J.C. and Pharm, D., "Medication Errors: Picking up the Pieces," *Drug Topics*, March 1999, pp. 83–92.

8. Phillips, D.P., Christenfeld, N., and Glynn, L.M., "Increase in US Medication-error Deaths Between 1983 and 1993," *Lancet*, Vol. 351, 1998, pp. 643–644.

9. *Industry Profile and Healthcare Factbook*, National Wholesale Druggists' Association, Reston, Virginia, 1998.

10. Wechsler, J., "Manufacturers Challenged to Reduce Medication Errors," *Pharmaceutical Technology*, February 2000, pp. 14–22.

11. Smith, D.L., "Medication Errors and DTC Ads.," *Pharmaceutical Executive*, February 2000, pp. 129–130.

12. Webster, S.A., "Technology Helps Reduce Mistakes on Medications," *The Detroit News*, February 6, 2000.

13. Roughead, E.E., Gilbert, A.L., Primrose, J.G., *et al.*, "Drug-Related Hospital Admissions: A Review of Australian Studies Published 1988–1996," *Medical Journal Australia*, Vol. 168, 1998, pp. 405–408.

14. Sullivan, S.D., Kreling, D.H., Hazlet, T.K., *et al.*, "Noncompliance with Medication Regimens and Subsequent Hospitalizations: A Literature Analysis and Cost of Hospitalization Estimate," *J. Research in Pharmaceutical Economics*, Vol. 2, No. 2, 1990, pp. 19–33.

15. Conlan, M.F., "IOM's Medical-Error Report Spurs Changes Among Pharmacies," *Drug Topics*, Vol. 144, 2000, pp. 70–71.

16. Domizio, G.D., Davis, N.M., and Cohen, M.R., "The Growing Risk of Lookalike Trademarks," *Medical Marketing and Media*, May 1992, pp. 24–30.

17. Ferner, R.E., "Medication Errors that Have Led to Manslaughter Charges," *British Medical Journal*, Vol. 321, 2000, pp. 1212–1216.

18. "Doctor Jailed for Attempting to Cover Up Fatal Error," *Guardian* (a UK Newspaper), May 7, 1994, p. 8.

19. Bindler, R. and Bayne, T., "Medication Calculation Ability of Registered Nurses," *IMAGE*, Vol. 23, No. 4, 1991, pp. 221–224.

20. Stewart, M.L., "Toxic Risks of Inappropriate Therapy," *Clinical Biochemistry*, Vol. 23, 1990, pp. 73–77.

21. "ASHP Guidelines on Preventing Medication Errors in Hospitals," *American Journal of Hospital Pharmacology*, Vol. 50, 1993, pp. 305–314.

22. Fox, G.N., "Minimizing Prescribing Errors in Infants and Children," *American Family Physician*, Vol. 53, No. 4, 1996, pp. 1319–1325.

23. O'Shea, E., "Factor Contributing to Medication Errors: A Literature Review," *Journal of Clinical Nursing*, Vol. 8, 1999, pp. 496–504.
24. Lilley, L.L. and Guanci, R., "Unfamiliar Drug Uses," *American Journal of Nursing*, Vol. 95, No. 1, 1995, pp. 18–19.
25. Leape, L.L., Bates, D.W., Cullen, D.J., *et al.*, "Systems Analysis of Adverse Drug Events," *JAMA*, Vol. 274, No. 1, 1995, pp. 35–43.
26. Bindler, R. and Bayne, T., "Do Baccalaureate Students Possess Basic Mathematics Proficiency?," *Journal of Nursing Education*, Vol. 23, No. 5, 1984, pp. 192–197.
27. Bayne, T. and Bindler, R., "Medication Calculation Skills of Registered Nurses," *Journal of Continuing Education in Nursing*, Vol. 19, No. 6, 1988, pp. 258–262.
28. Gold, D.R., Rogacz, S., Bock, N., *et al.*, "Rotating Shift Work, Sleep, and Accident Related to Sleepiness in Hospital Nurses," *American Journal of Public Health*, Vol. 82, No. 7, 1992, pp. 1011–1014.
29. Girotti, M.J., Garrick, C., Tierney, M.G., *et al.*, "Medication Administration Errors in an Adult Intensive Care Unit," *Heart and Lung*, Vol. 16, No. 4, 1987, pp. 449–453.
30. Conklin, D., MacFarland, V., Kinnie-Steeves, A., and Chenger, P., "Medication Errors by Nurses: Contributing Factors," *AARN Newsletter*, Vol. 46, No. 1, 1990, pp. 8–9.
31. Fuqua, R.A. and Stevens, K.R., "What We Know About Medication Errors: A Literature Review," *Journal of Nursing Quality Assurance*, Vol. 3, No. 1, 1988, pp. 1–17.
32. Jeanes, A. and Taylor, D., "Stopping the Drugs Trolley," *Nursing Times*, Vol. 88, No. 2, 1992, pp. 27–29.
33. Kruse, H., Johnson, A., O'Connell, D., and Clarke, T., "Administering Restricted Medications in Hospital: The Implications and Costs of Using Two Nurses," *Australian Clinical Review*, Vol. 12, No. 2, 1992, pp. 77–83.
34. Long, G. and Johnson, C., "A Pilot Study for Reducing Medication Errors," *Quality Review Bulletin*, Vol. 7, No. 4, 1981, pp. 6–9.
35. Howell, M., "Prescription for Disaster," *Nursing Times*, Vol. 92, No. 34, 1996, pp. 30–31.
36. Davis, N.M., "Concentrating on Interruptions," *American Journal of Nursing*, Vol. 94, No. 3, 1994, pp. 14–15.
37. Bates, D.W., Teich, J., Lee, J., *et al.*, "The Impact of Computerized Physician Order Entry on Medication Error Prevention," *Journal of American Medical Informatics Association*, Vol. 6, 1999, pp. 313–321.
38. Classen, D.C., Pestotnik, S.L., Evans, R.S., and Burke, J.P., "Computerized Surveillance of Adverse Drug Events in Hospital Patients," *JAMA*, Vol. 266, 1991, pp. 2847–2851.
39. Jha, A.K., Kuperman, G.J., Teich, J.M., *et al.*, "Identifying Adverse Drug Events: Development of a Computer-based Monitor and Comparison to Chart Review and Stimulated Voluntary Report," *Journal of American Medical Informatics Association*, Vol. 5, 1998, pp. 305–314.

40. Barker, K.N., "Ensuring Safety in the Use of Automated Medication Dispensing Systems," *Am. J. Health Syst. Pharm.*, Vol. 35, 1995, pp. 25–33.
41. Boral, J.M. and Rascati, K.L., "Effect of an Automated, Nursing Unit-based Drug-Dispensing Device on Medication Errors," *Am. J. Health Syst. Pharm.*, Vol. 52, 1995, pp. 1875–1879.
42. Knox, R., "Prescription Errors Tied to Lack of Advice: Pharmacists Skirting Law," *Massachusetts Study*, Boston Globe, February 10, 1999, p. B1.
43. Wilson, D.G., McArtney, R.G., Newcombe, R.G., *et al.*, "Medication Errors in Pediatric Practice: Insights from a Continuous Quality Improvement Approach," *Eur. J. Pediatr.*, Vol. 157, 1998, pp. 769–774.
44. Bates, D.W., Boyle, D.L., Vander-Vilet, *et al.*, "Relationship between Medication Errors and Adverse Drug Events," *J. Gen. Intern. Med.*, Vol. 10, 1995, pp. 199–205.
45. Lesar, T.S., Briceland, L., and Stein, D.S., "Factors Related to Errors in Medication Prescribing," *JAMA*, Vol. 277, 1997, pp. 312–317.
46. Folli, H.L., Poole, R.L., Benitz, W.E., *et al.*, "Medication Error Prevention by Clinical Pharmacists in Two Children's Hospitals," *Pediatrics*, Vol. 79, 1987, pp. 718–722.

Chapter 7

Human Error in Anesthesia

7.1 Introduction

Anesthesiology may simply be described as the branch of the medical field that is concerned with the processes of rendering patients insensitive to various types of pain during surgery or when faced with chronic/acute pain states.[1] Furthermore, an anesthetized patient may simply be regarded as an individual who has been intentionally made critically ill. A person who administers anesthesia is known as an anesthetist and a physician specializing in anesthesiology is called an anesthesiologist.

The history of successful anesthetists may be traced back to Joseph Clover who up to 1871 administered around 7000 general anesthetics, with chloroform as an inhalational anaesthetic agent, without the occurrence of a single death.[2] Although the first anesthetic death was reported in 1848, it took a long time to realize that human error is an important factor in the occurrence of anesthesia-related deaths.[3,4]

Human error in anesthesia may be defined in two ways: a slip or a mistake.[5] A slip is an action (or lack of action) by the anesthetist/anesthesiologist that did not occur as planned. A mistake is a decision leading to an action or a lack of action by the anesthetist/anesthesiologist that is causally linked to an actual or probable adverse outcome. This chapter presents the various important aspects of human error in anesthesia.

7.2   Facts and Figures

Some of the facts and figures directly or indirectly concerned with human error in anesthesia are as follows:

- Each year between 2000 and 10000 patients in the United States alone die from anesthesia attributed reasons.[5,6]
- For the period from 1948 to 1952, the risk of death solely attributed to anesthesia was 1 in 2680.[7]
- From 1952 to 1984, the risk of death solely due to anesthesia has decreased from 1 in 2680 to around 1 in 10000.[8]
- A sample of 1147000 surgical operations performed in certain health care facilities indicates that out of the 6060 patients who died within six days after the surgery, 227 were partially or completely due to anesthesia.[6]
- A study of 163240 anesthetics given over a period of 15 years revealed that a total of 27 anesthetics-related cardiac arrests occurred. A further investigation of these cardiac arrests pointed out that the failure in providing sufficient ventilation caused almost half of the arrests and one third resulted from the absolute overdose of an inhalation agent.[9]
- In 80 anesthesia-related deaths, human error was believed to be responsible for 87% of the cases.[10,11]
- In 589 anesthesia-related deaths, human error was considered to be a factor in 83% of the cases.[10,12]
- In 52 anesthesia-related deaths, human error was believed to be responsible for 65% of the cases.[10,13]
- From 1970 to 1977, a total of 277 anesthetic-related deaths occurred and factors such as faulty technique (43%), coexistent disease (12%), the failure of postoperative care (10%), and drug overdose (5%) were considered responsible for the deaths.[8]
- A major Hong Kong teaching hospital administered 16000 anesthetics in one year and reported 125 related critical incidents, in which human error was an important factor (i.e. 80% of the cases).[14]

7.3   Frequent Anesthesia Errors and Their Causes and Modes of Human Error in Anesthesia

Over the years various studies have been performed to determine the frequent anesthesia errors and their common causes. Tables 7.1 and 7.2 present some of the most common anesthesia errors and their frequent causes,

Table 7.1. Common anesthesia errors.

No.	Error
1	Syringe swap
2	Breathing circuit disconnection
3	Drug overdose
4	Ventilator failure
5	Breathing circuit leak
6	Premature extubation
7	Breathing circuit misconnection
8	Incorrect blood transfused
9	Loss of oxygen supply
10	Ampule swap
11	Unintentional extubation
12	Inadvertent change in gas flow
13	Incorrect selection of airway management method
14	Endobronchial intubation
15	Hypoventilation (operator error)

Table 7.2. Some frequent causes of anesthesia errors.

No.	Cause
1	Poor anesthesia-related experience
2	Fatigue and haste
3	Failure to carry out a proper checkout/history
4	Poor familiarity with anesthetic method
5	Poor familiarity with surgical procedure
6	Carelessness
7	Inadequate communication with the surgical team, or the laboratory personnel
8	Emergency case
9	Poor familiarity with equipment device
10	Excessive reliance on other personnel
11	Teaching activity in progress
12	Lack of skilled assistance or supervision
13	Visual field restricted

respectively.[6,15] In fact, some of these studies have ranked the occurrence frequency of the anesthesia errors and the frequency of their causes (i.e. highest to lowest), for example, Tables 7.3 and 7.4 present the result of two such studies.[16,17]

Table 7.3.   Anesthesia errors in two distinct studies A[16] and B[17] ranked according to the frequency of their occurrence (i.e. highest to lowest).

Rank	Study A: Error	Study B: Error
1(highest)	Breathing circuit disconnection during mechanical ventilation	Breathing circuit disconnection
2	Syringe swap	Inadvertent gas flow change
3	Gas flow control (technical error)	Syringe swap
4	Loss of gas supply	Gas supply problem
5	Disconnection of intravenous line	Disconnection of intravenous apparatus
6	Vaporizer off unintentionally	Laryngoscope failure
7	Drug ampule swap	Premature extubation
8	Drug overdose (syringe, judgmental)	Hypovolemia
9	Drug overdose (vaporizer, technical)	Tracheal airway device position changes
10	Breathing circuit leak	—
11	Unintentional extubation	—
12	Misplaced tracheal tube	—
13	Breathing circuit misconnection	—
14	Inadequate fluid replacement	—
15	Premature extubation	—
16	Ventilator failure	—
17	Improper use of blood pressure monitor	—
18	Breathing-circuit control technical error	—
19	Incorrect selection of airway management method	—
20	Laryngoscope failure	—
21	Incorrect IV line used	—
22	Hypoventilation	—
23	Drug overdose (vaporizer, judgmental	—
24	Drug overdose (syringe, technical)	—
25 (lowest)	Incorrect drug selection	—

Table 7.4. Anesthesia error causes in two distinct studies A[16] and B[17] ranked according to the frequency of their occurrence (i.e. highest to lowest).

Rank	Study A: Error cause	Study B: Error cause
1 (highest)	Failure to check	Poor total experience
2	Very first experience with situation	Poor familiarity with equipment
3	Poor total experience	Inadequate communication with team, laboratory people, etc.
4	Carelessness	Carelessness
5	Haste	Haste
6	Unfamiliarity with equipment	Over dependency on other people
7	Visual restriction	Fatigue
8	Poor familiarity with anesthesia method	Failure to carry out a normal check
9	Distractive simultaneous anesthesia activities	Training/experience
10	Over dependency on other people	Lack of supervisor's presence
11	Teaching in progress	Environment/colleagues
12	Unfamiliarity with surgical procedure	Visual restriction
13	Fatigue	Mental/physical
14	Lack of supervisor's presence	Poor experience with surgical process
15	Failure to follow personal routine	Distraction
16	Poor supervision	Inadequate labeling of controls, drugs, etc.
17	Conflicting equipment designs	Supervision
18	Unfamiliarity with drug	Situations precluded normal precautions
19	Failure to follow institutional practices and procedures effectively	Poor familiarity with anesthetic method
20	—	Teaching activity in action
21	—	Apprehension
22	—	Emergency situation
23	—	Difficult/demanding case
24	—	Boredom
25	—	Nature of activity
26	—	Inadequate preparation
27 (lowest)	—	Slow procedure

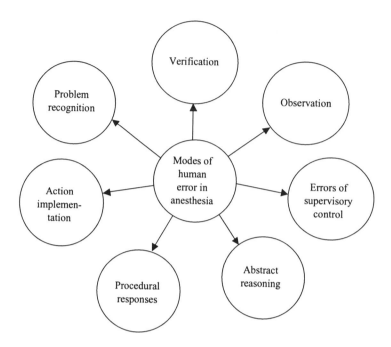

Fig. 7.1.   Basic modes of human error in anesthesia with respect to decision making.

More specifically, Tables 7.3 and 7.4 have ranked the anesthesia errors and their causes, respectively, from the highest to the lowest occurrence frequency.

There are basically seven modes of human error in anesthesia with respect to decision making as shown in Fig. 7.1.[5] These are problem recognition, observation, verification, abstract reasoning, procedural responses, action implementation, and errors of supervisory control.

The sub-elements of problem recognition are: the true observation not recognized as abnormal, and the wrong "problem" recognized (i.e. misdiagnosis). Three sub-elements of observation are: misperception, data stream not available, and data stream not checked frequent enough (i.e. because of vigilance failure due to excessive work load, vigilance failure due to human performance factors (e.g. fatigue), and vigilance failure due to the lack of diligence). The verification mode has two sub-elements: incorrect data used in decision-making, and actions taken on unverified false positive. The sub-elements of abstract reasoning are: incomplete or wrong medical knowledge, logic error, insufficient hypotheses generated, calculation error, inadequate or erroneous data requested, and missing or erroneous therapeutic options.

Two sub-elements of the procedural responses are: right problem, incorrect procedure, and right problem, right but incomplete procedure. The action implementation mode has three sub-elements: improper method, unavailable tool or drug and slips (e.g. memory error, description error, and sequence error). The sub-elements of the errors of supervisory control mode are: data steam selection, prioritization (e.g. ignoring true positive, excessive priority given to one problem, or insufficient priority given to recognized problem), re-evaluation (i.e. fixation errors (e.g. "This and only this" or "everything but this"), the failure to re-check critical data, considering a single problem with multiple manifestations, considering multiple simultaneous problems, and abandoning ineffective actions), and action planning (i.e. the failure to consider constraints, delay, side effects, preconditions, reversibility, ease of implementation, and certainty of success).

The above seven modes of human error also correspond to the components of the anesthesiologist's decision making model which will be discussed in the next section.

7.4 Anesthesiologist Decision Making Model

This model assumes that an anesthesiologist works at four abstraction levels: sensory/motor level ("skill-based"), procedural level ("rule-based"), abstract level ("knowledge-based"), and the supervisory control level.[5] The sensory/motor level is concerned with the processing of sensory data and the control of motor actions. The procedural level is concerned with responding to problems as indicated in the stored rules or the precompiled routines. The abstract level is concerned with responding to problems by abstract manipulation of concepts and logical propositions. The supervisory control level is concerned with procedures such as coordinating attention between levels, allocating attention between different problems or different set of actions, and coordinating interactions between the anesthesiologist and the "outside world".

The model has many specific components that require a careful consideration with respect to the abstraction levels. The specific model components are as follows[5]:

- **Observation.** As the intervention of an accident starts with data observation, the anesthesiologist establishes "streams" of data to be sampled, including the visual observation of the patient, the surgical area, and the various monitor displays and auditory channels. In situations when the anesthesiologist does not make frequent observations, or when useful data streams are not available (e.g. precordial/esophageal stethoscope is not used), or if there is a faulty perception, errors may occur.

- **Procedural responses.** An anesthesiologist's initial response to a problem must be fast and efficient. More specifically, there must be well established procedures for guiding the anesthesiologist in emergency situations. Errors associated with procedural responses include retrieving the incorrect responses for the correct problem as well as committing an error within a generally proper response plan.

- **Observation verification.** In most observations made during anesthesia, there is an element of uncertainty. Moreover, unlike industrial workers having well instrumented systems, anesthesiologists apply largely external instruments to patients and then remove the devices only at the end of the specified procedure. Due to such limitations, the data verification process is very important, otherwise, a catastrophe may result, particularly, when a real problem is ignored or a non-existent one is treated inappropriately.

- **Abstract reasoning.** Past experiences indicate that some problems can be unfamiliar or unaffected by standardized responses. From time to time, even the solved problems require further understanding so that they can be prevented or treated specifically in the future.[18] Situations such as these require an abstract reasoning to a certain degree, for example, by forming a hypothesis and then testing it using new or existing data. Errors in abstract reasoning can occur if incorrect or incomplete knowledge is provided or if the correct hypothesis is not included initially.

- **Action implementation.** As success is not automatically guaranteed by merely selecting the appropriate course of action, the effective implementation of the action is an equally important factor in this aspect. For example, the implementation of actions using a faulty method is likely to reduce the rate of success. Moreover, from time to time errors do occur even during practiced actions.

- **Problem recognition and assessment.** An observation can be interpreted either as normal or abnormal. In the case of abnormality, an explanation is sought after and its severity is weighed relative to the other events (i.e. prioritization). A frequent error is the misdiagnosing of an abnormality.[5]

- **Supervisory control.** An anesthesiologist's attention must be divided to three main areas: data collection, problem solving and manual tasking. The coordination of the different cognitive levels (i.e. thinking versus doing) and the management of various problems simultaneously are important components of dynamic decision-making. The main areas, with respect to supervisory control, in which an anesthesiologist frequently makes mistakes are namely: data stream selection, prioritization, re-evaluation, and action planning.

Figure 7.1 presents the modes of human error corresponding to the above seven model components.

7.5 Methods for Preventing or Reducing Anesthetic Mishaps with Respect to Human Error

Over the years many different methods or strategies have been proposed for preventing or reducing anesthetic mishaps. As these methods consist of a number of steps or elements, they may overlap to a certain degree. This section presents three such methods.

7.5.1 *Method I*

This method is quite useful for preventing errors as well as detecting those errors and system failures that may slip through the first line of defense. This method is composed of seven elements as shown in Fig. 7.2.[5] The element "train and supervise" is concerned with providing an appropriate level

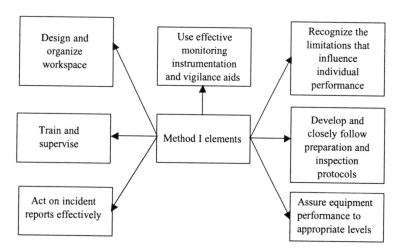

Fig. 7.2. Method I elements.

of training in technical skills, factual knowledge, or the use of equipment and devices, as well as assuring the availability of appropriate amount of supervision and guidance.[19,20]

The element "design and organize work space" is concerned with designing and organizing of an effective work space by considering the people, the equipment, and the tasks associated with anesthesia so that the probability of error occurrence is reduced and the accuracy and the speed of response are improved. The element "use effective monitoring instrumentation and vigilance aids" is concerned with the use of effective monitoring instrumentation and vigilance aids so that the occurrence of human error is minimized.

The element "recognize the limitations that influence individual performance" is concerned with realizing the factors that influence individual performance directly or indirectly. Some examples of these factors are: personal stress and life change events, fatigue and the scheduling of work-rest cycles, as well as excessive haste.[21,22] More specifically, factors such as these may play an important role in the occurrence of anesthesia-related human errors. The element "develop and closely follow preparation and inspection protocols" is concerned with the establishment and close adherence of effective preparation and inspection protocols since various past studies indicate that poor preparation for anesthesia or surgery contribute to at least 53% of the fatal mishaps. The failure to carry out a thorough check of equipment used was singled out as the most frequent factor associated with critical incidents.

The element "assure equipment performance to appropriate levels" is concerned with assuring anesthesia-associated equipment performance by considering carefully factors such as preventive maintenance, peruse inspection, and the recognition of obsolescence. The element "act on incident report effectively" is concerned with taking appropriate corrective measures with regards to the findings of incident reports so that the potential problems are eradicated altogether.

7.5.2   *Method II*

This is another method of preventing or reducing anesthetic mishaps with respect to human error. The method consists of the following steps[23]:

- **Discover what is going on.** This is concerned with determining the existing state of affairs. This can be determined by reviewing items such as medical defense reports, mortality committee reports, morbidity committee reports, hazard alerts, incident monitoring studies, observation studies, and simulation studies.

- **Collate the information.** This is concerned with collating information and collecting subsets for studies and classifications. This calls for the establishment of a project team as well as having adequate access to the appropriate information. A team can be made up of any groups, say, a department in charge of addressing a specific problem. More specifically, an example of a team is the confidential morbidity and/or the mortality review committee.

- **Classify problem errors and contributing factors.** This is concerned with the grouping of errors, problems, and contributing factors into the appropriate classifications.

- **Develop appropriate preventative strategies.** This is concerned with detecting, preventing, avoiding, and minimizing the potential consequences. From time to time, the problems with a complex set of contributing factors may require the development of preventive strategies at several levels. All in all, proper care must be given to ensure that the strategies are as practical as possible for their successful implementation.

- **Implement strategies.** This is basically concerned with putting strategies into appropriate places. Effective communication plays a key role in the implementation of strategies.

- **Review strategies in action.** This is concerned with assessing the effective functioning of strategies and enforcing the appropriate corrective measures (if warranted).

7.5.3   *Method III*

This methods calls for action in the five distinct areas as shown in Fig. 7.3 to minimize the occurrence of anesthesia-related human errors. These five areas are: organization, supervision, education, equipment, and protocols.[14] There are two important actions associated with organization, namely: improving communication between all staff personnel as well as revising work policies to reduce haste or stress. Actions such as ensuring complete pre-operative assessments of patients as well as ensuring available supervision and additional help if required, are associated with the supervision area.

The education area calls for the review of reported incidents on a regular basis as well as upgrading all operating room staff through courses

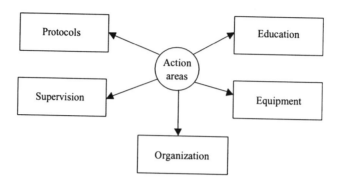

Fig. 7.3.   Areas for action to reduce the occurrence of human error in anesthesia.

and seminars. There are three equipment-related actions, namely: adopt appropriate measures to check equipment prior to its use, replace faulty or inappropriate pieces, and provide adequate number and types of monitors. The protocols area calls for the formulation of protocols for repetitive tasks, patient monitoring, and patient transport.

7.6   Anesthesia Error-Related Studies*

Over the years many anesthesia error-related studies have been performed. Some of these studies are directly or indirectly related to anesthesia error and they are discussed below.

- **Cooper *et al.* Study.**[10] In this study 47 interviews of staff and resident anesthesiologists from a large urban teaching hospital for the period from September 1975 to April 1977 were conducted with respect to preventable anesthesia mishaps. A total of 359 preventable critical incidents were identified and 82% involved human error to a certain degree.
- **Dripps *et al.* Study.**[11] This study reviewed records of 33224 patients anesthetized in a 10-year period. The study revealed that 12 of the 18737 patients following the application of spinal anesthesia died due to anesthesia-related causes and 27 of the 14487 patients following the receipt of a general anesthesia supplemented with a muscle relaxant died from causes directly-related to anesthesia.

---

*Some material presented in this section may directly or indirectly overlap with certain contents in Sec. 7.2.

- **Beecher and Todd Study.**[7] This study reviewed the records of all deaths due to surgical services of ten University hospitals from January 1948 to December 1952. The study revealed that 7977 of the 599548 patients died after receiving anesthesia and 29 of the 384 deaths caused by anesthesia were the result of gross errors.
- **Morris and Morris Study.**[24] This study reviewed the Australian Incident Monitoring Study (AIMS) database of the Australian Patient Safety Foundation (APSF) for the period of April 1987 to October 1997. During this period a total of 5600 reports were reviewed and 152 were considered fatigue-positive reports or in which fatigue was listed as a factor contributing to the incidents. A further examination of the fatigue-positive reports revealed that the incidents were more frequent during the induction phase of the anesthesia and they are less frequent during maintenance.
- **McDonald and Peterson Study.**[25] This study surveyed 287 private practitioners with respect to operating room accidents during anesthesia. The analysis of the survey revealed that around 23% of the respondents admitted to having committed a lethal error ever before.
- **Craig and Wilson Study.**[15] This study examined 8312 anesthetics administered in the Anesthetic Department of a general hospital over a 6-month period. The study revealed a total of 81 anesthetic misadventures. A further examination of these misadventures revealed that human error was more often responsible for these misadventures rather than equipment failure, and the failure to conduct regular checks was the factor most frequently associated with these misadventures.
- **Chopra *et al.* Study.**[26] This study was performed at a teaching hospital over an 18-month period with respect to anesthesia-related problems. The study reported a total of 549 significant incidents and out which 411 were considered to be attributed to human error.

Problems

1. Define the term "human error in anesthesia".
2. List at least eight facts and figures concerned with human error in anesthesia.
3. List at least fifteen common anesthesia errors.
4. What are the causes for the occurrence of anesthesia errors?

5. Discuss the modes of human error in anesthesia with respect to decision making.
6. Discuss the anesthesiologist decision-making model.
7. Discuss the methods of preventing or reducing anesthetic mishaps with respect to human error.
8. Discuss at least five anesthesia error-related studies.
9. Define the term "anesthesiology".
10. List the top five anesthesia errors in the order of their occurrence frequency (i.e. highest to lowest).

References

1. Gaba, D.M., "Human Error in Dynamic Medical Domains," in *Human Error in Medicine*, M.S. Bogner (ed), Lawrence Erlbaum Associates, Publishers, Hillsdale, New Jersey, 1994, pp. 197–223.
2. Roelofse, J.A. and Shipton, E.A., "Obstruction of a Breathing Circuit: A Case Report," *South African Medical Journal*, Vol. 66, No. 13, 1984, pp. 501–502.
3. Beecher, H.K., "The First Anesthesia Death with Some Remarks Suggested by it on the Fields of the Laboratory and the Clinic in the Appraisal of New Anesthetic Agents," *Anesthesiology*, Vol. 2, 1941, pp. 443–449.
4. Cooper, J.B., Newbower, R.S., and Kitz, R.J., "An Analysis of Major Errors and Equipment Failures in Anesthesia Management: Considerations for Prevention and Detection," *Anesthesiology*, Vol. 60, 1984, pp. 34–42.
5. Gaba, D.M., "Human Error in Anesthetic Mishaps," *International Anesthesiology Clinics*, Vol. 27, No. 3, 1989, pp. 137–147.
6. Cooper, J.B., "Toward Prevention of Anesthetic Mishaps," *International Anesthesiology Clinics*, Vol. 22, 1984, pp. 167–183.
7. Beecher, H.K. and Todd, D.P., "A Study of the Deaths Associated with Anethesia and Surgery Based on a Study of 599548 Anethesia in ten Institutions 1948–1952, Inclusive," *Annals of Surgery*, Vol. 140, 1954, pp. 2–35.
8. Davies, J.M. and Strunin, L., "Anethesia in 1984: How Safe Is It?," *Canadian Medical Association Journal*, Vol. 131, September 1984, pp. 437–441.
9. Keenan, R.L. and Boyan, C.P., "Cardiac Arrest Due to Anesthesia," *The Journal of the American Medical Association (JAMA)*, Vol. 253, No. 16, 1985, pp. 2373–2377.
10. Cooper, J.B., Newbower, R.S., Long, C.D., *et al.*, "Preventable Anesthesia Mishaps," *Anesthesiology*, Vol. 49, 1978, pp. 399–406.
11. Dripps, R.D., Lamont, A., and Eckenhoff, J.E., "The Role of Anesthesia in Surgical Mortality," *JAMA*, Vol. 178, 1961, pp. 261–266.
12. Edwards, G., Morton, H.J.V., and Pask, E.A., "Deaths Associated with Anesthesia: Report on 1000 Cases," *Anesthesia*, Vol. 11, 1956, pp. 194–220.

13. Clifton, B.S. and Hotten, W.I.T., "Deaths Associated with Anesthesia," *British Journal of Anesthesia*, Vol. 35, 1963, pp. 250–259.
14. Short, T.G., O'Regan, A., Lew, J., and Oh, T.E., "Critical Incident Reporting in an Anesthetic Department Quality Assurance Program," *Anesthesia*, Vol. 47, 1992, pp. 3–7.
15. Craig, J. and Wilson, M.E., "A Survey of Anesthetic Misadventures," *Anesthesia*, Vol. 36, 1981, pp. 933–938.
16. Cooper, J.B., Newbower, R.S., and Kitz, R.J., "An Analysis of Major Errors and Equipment Failures in Anesthesia Management: Considerations for Prevention and Detection," *Anesthesiology*, Vol. 60, 1984, pp. 34–42.
17. Cooper, J.B., Newbower, R.S., Long, C.D., *et al.*, "Preventable Anesthesia Mishaps: A Study of Human Factors," *Anesthesiology*, Vol. 49, 1978, pp. 399–406.
18. Woods, D.D., "Coping with Complexity: The Psychology of Human Behavior in Complex Systems," in *Tasks, Errors, and Mental Models*, L.P. Goodstein, H.B. Andersen, and S.E. Olsen (eds), Taylor and Francis, 1988, pp. 128–148.
19. Levin, M.J. and Balasaraswathi, K., "Fail Safe? Unsafe!," *Anesthesiology*, Vol. 48, 1978, pp. 152–153.
20. Lunn, J.N. and Mushin, W.W., *Mortality Associated with Anesthesia*, Report, Nuffield Provincial Hospital Trust, London, Ontario, 1982.
21. Selzer, M.L., Roges, J.E., and Kern, S., "Fatal Accidents: The Role of Psychopathology, Social Stress and Acute Disturbance," *American Journal of Psychiatry*, Vol. 124, 1968, pp. 124–126.
22. Sheehan, D.V., O'Donnel, J., Fitzgerald, A., *et al.*, "Psychosocial Predictors of Accident/Error Rates in Nursing Students: A Prospective Study," *International Journal of Psychiatry Medicine*, Vol. 11, 1981, pp. 125–128.
23. Runciman, W.B., Sellen, A., Webb, R.K., *et al.*, "Errors, Incidents and Accidents in Anesthetic Practice," *Anesthesia and Intensive Care*, Vol. 21, No. 5, 1993, pp. 506–518.
24. Morris, G.P. and Morris, R.W., "Anesthesia and Fatigue: An Analysis of the First 10 years of the Australian Incident Monitoring Study 1987–1997," *Anesthesia and Intensive Care*, Vol. 28, No. 3, 2000, pp. 300–303.
25. McDonald, J.S. and Peterson, S., "Lethal Errors in Anesthesiology," *Anesthesiology*, Vol. 63, No. 3A, 1985, pp. A497.
26. Chopra, V., Bovill, J.G., Spierdijk, J., *et al.*, "Reported Significant Observations During Anesthesia: A Prospective Analysis Over an 18-Month Period," *British Journal of Anesthesia*, Vol. 68, 1992, pp. 13–17.

Chapter 8

Human Error in Miscellaneous Health Care Areas and Health Care Human Error Cost

8.1 Introduction

Human error in health care is the eighth leading cause of deaths in the United States. In turn, many components and tasks are associated with the health care system (including intensive care units, emergency departments, test laboratories, operating rooms), in providing medication, administering anesthetics, taking laboratory samples, performing diagnosis, and interpreting images. Human error can occur in any one of these health care system components or units when various types of tasks are performed. For example, in an emergency department, with its myriad activities and extreme time demands, 93% of adverse events are considered preventable.[1,2] This is further reinforced by the fact that around 20% of the money awarded in malpractice suits against emergency department practitioners or doctors are concerned with the misdiagnosis and mistreatment of coronary syndromes.[3]

The cost of human errors in health care in the United States is astronomical. For example, as presented in Ref. 4, the total national cost of adverse events is around $38 billion and $17 billion of this amount is associated with preventable adverse events. Furthermore, as indicated in Ref. 5, the annual adverse drug events' cost alone in a hospital is estimated to be around $5.6 million and $2.8 million of this figure is accounted for by preventable adverse drug events. This chapter discusses the occurrence of human error in various health care areas as well as the health care human error-related costs.

8.2   Human Error in Intensive Care Units

Originally, intensive care started with the concentration of very ill, postoperative patients in a single room of a hospital where their condition could be monitored closely. By 1960, only 10% of the hospitals in the United States with over 200 beds had intensive care units, but by 1981, the percentage had increased to 99%.[6,7] Furthermore, during the same period the number of beds in the intensive care units increased quite significantly. For example, in the late 1970s the annual increase in the intensive care beds was around 4%.[6] Today, over 40000 patients nation-wide are warded in intensive care units each day, receiving various types of medical services. The performance of these services is subjected to human error. Nonetheless, some of the facts and figures directly or indirectly concerned with human error in intensive care units are as follows:

- A study of critical incident reports in an intensive care unit over a ten year period (i.e. 1989–1999) revealed that most of the incidents were due to staff errors and not due to equipment failures.[8]
- A study of human errors in an 11-bed multidisciplinary intensive care unit conducted over a twelve month period revealed that a total of 241 human errors occurred: one was lethal, two resulted in sequelae, 26% resulted in prolonged stay in the intensive care unit, 57% were minor, and only 16% was free of any consequence.[9]
- A study concerned with the nature and causes of human errors in a 6-bed intensive care unit conducted over a six-month period revealed that out of a total of 554 human errors reported by the medical staff,[10] 29% were considered severe or potentially detrimental to the patients. 45% of the total errors were committed by physicians and the remaining 55% by nurses.
- A study of seven intensive care units conducted over one year revealed that a total of 610 incidents occurred.[11] 66% of these incidents were due to human factor-related problems and the remaining 34% due to system-related problems.
- A study of 145 reports of adverse events, involving patients in an intensive care unit during the period from 1974 to 1978, presented 92 cases of human error and 53 cases of equipment failure.[12]
- A study of pharmacist participation on physician rounds and adverse drug events in the intensive care unit reported that the presence of a pharmacist on duty as a full member of the patient care team in an

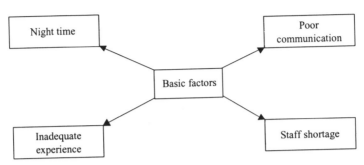

Fig. 8.1.   Four basic factors for the occurrence of human errors in intensive care units.

intensive care unit helps to reduce substantially the occurrence of adverse drug events due to prescribing errors.[13]

Researchers working in the area of analyzing the occurrence of human errors in intensive care units have identified a number of error contributing factors. Four such factors are shown in Fig. 8.1.[8]

With respect to the detection of incidents in intensive care units, some of the contributing factors are: regular checking, the presence of properly experienced staff, and the presence of alarms on the equipment.

8.3   Human Error in Emergency Medicine

The emergency departments are subjected to the occurrence of human error just like any other medical departments. As there are around 100 million emergency department patient visits annually in the United States, even a minute percentage of human error occurrence can translate to a substantial number of related adverse events.[14] Some of the facts and figures directly or indirectly concerned with the emergency medicine are as follows:

- In emergency departments, over 90% of the adverse events are considered preventable.[2,15]
- In the interpretation of radiographs, the rates of disagreement between emergency physicians and radiologists vary from 8–11%.[16]
- A study concerned with determining the rate of error in emergency physician interpretation of the cause of electro-cardiographic (ECG) ST-Segment elevation (STE) in adult chest pain patients reported that out of the 202 patients who had STEs, the rate of ECG STE misinterpretation was approximately 6%.[17]

- A study of missed diagnoses of acute cardiac ischemia in an emergency department revealed that out of the 1817 patients with acute cardiac ischemia approximately 4.3% were mistakenly discharged from the emergency department.[18]

To prevent the occurrence of human errors in emergency medicine, it is important to accurately assess the possible risk or the predictor factors. Therefore from the public health standpoint, epidemiological methods and techniques should be employed to highlight the causes of emergency medicine errors and their resulting adverse events.[18–20] Questions such as those listed below can directly or indirectly help to reduce the occurrence of human errors in emergency medicine[18]:

- Is it possible to make human errors more visible when they occur?
- Are the computerized clinical information systems helpful in reducing the occurrence of human errors and their associated adverse events in the emergency department setting?
- What is the effects of lowering health care provider distractions on the occurrence of human error in emergency medicine? Two examples of such distractions are telephone calls and paging interruptions.
- Are there any ideal lengths of shifts and change-of-shift approaches for lowering the occurrence of human error in emergency medicine?
- Does the presence of a pharmacologist help to reduce the occurrence of human errors and adverse events in the emergency department setting?

8.4   Human Error in Operating Rooms

The effectiveness of team performance in the operating room is very important as surgical tasks require the coordinated effects of professionals such as doctors and nurses working under time pressure. A human error in such an environment can result in death or permanent damage to a patient. In turn, this may lead to various types of legal actions. Nonetheless, professionals such as those listed below form the operating room teams.[21]

- Surgeons.
- Anesthetists.
- Surgical nurses.
- Anesthetic nurses.
- Individuals from the support services.

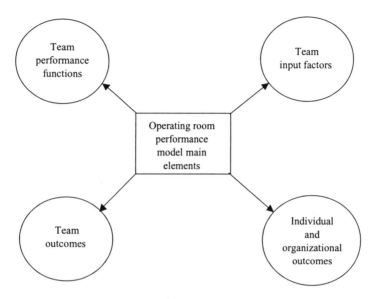

Fig. 8.2.   Main elements of the model of operating room performance.

Although the size of an operating room team depends on factors such as the complexity of the operation and the condition of the patient, it usually varies from 4 to 15 people.[22] Commission and omission errors can occur in the operating room environment, and some examples of these errors are: severing an artery or administering an inappropriate drug, and failing to note falling blood pressure, respectively.

In order to investigate the occurrence of human error in the operating room effectively, it is essential to understand a model representing the operating room performance. The main elements of the model of the operating room performance are shown in Fig. 8.2,[21] namely: team input factors, team performance functions, team outcomes, and individual and organizational outcomes. The team input factors include individual aptitudes, team composition, time pressure, personality/motivation, patient condition, physical condition, and organizational climate/norms. Teams performance faction associated elements are: team formation, team management, communication skills, technical procedures, conflict resolution, situational awareness, and decision processes. Team outcome factors include patient safety and team efficiency. Individual and organizational outcome related elements are: attitudes, morale, and professional development.

The study of this model directly or indirectly highlights the fact that there are many instances which can lead to the occurrence of human error in the operating room. Some of the observed problems in operating room team coordination are as follows:

- Failure to establish good leadership for the operating team.
- Failure to plan patient preparation effectively, anticipate surgeon actions, and monitor other team activities in an effective manner.
- Failure to debrief operation to learn from past situations for future reference.
- Failure to brief one's own team and the other teams when planning for an operation.
- Failure to discuss alternative procedures and advocate own position effectively and to inform team members of work overload or patient related problems.
- Unresolved differences between surgical team and anesthetists.
- Frustrations due to poor team coordination.
- Consultants' failure to provide adequate training to residents.

Human errors observed in the operating room from the behavioral aspect can be categorized into the following three classifications[21]:

- **Classification I:** Preparation/planning/vigilance.
- **Classification II:** Communications/decisions.
- **Classification III:** Workload distribution/distraction avoidance.

Some examples of Classification I errors are: failure to monitor patient status during operation, failure to react to blood pressure and blood oxygen alarms, failure to complete checklist (e.g. anesthesia machine set incorrectly), and failure to anticipate events during a complex procedure (e.g. coming off coronary bypass).

Examples such as the failure of the surgeon to inform the anesthetist of drugs having effects on blood pressure, the consultant drawing up patient schedules without appropriately informing the resident or the nursing staff, and the consultant leaving work overloaded resident staff in the operating room all belong to the Classification II errors.

Two examples of Classification III errors are: the consultant being distracted from making a decision to place a pulmonary artery catheter by problems identified by another operating facility, and the resident staff reading the technical manual, distracted from that the patient is not adequately relaxed.

8.5   Human Error in Image Interpretation, Laboratory Testing, Medical Technology Use, and Radiotherapy

The misinterpretation of medical results such as X-ray, electro-cardiograms, CAT scan, and sonograms is a common cause of diagnostic errors.[22–23] Past experiences indicate that image misinterpretation problem is often related to inexperienced and junior doctors.[22–24] Nonetheless, currently research is being performed to explore various aspects of the image interpretation process that may lead to improvements in image interpretation performance.[22,25]

Over the years, various types of human errors in laboratory testing have been reported. For example, the New York State laboratory regulators discovered testing errors in approximately 66% of the laboratories offering drug-screening services.[22,26] It means that there is a definite need for an effective laboratory testing system to minimize the occurrence of human errors.

Over the years, with the increase in sophistication and the complexity of medical technology, human errors in medical technology have increased significantly.[22,27] Some of the factors for the occurrence of errors are: the poor standardization of devices, inadequate or no consideration to human factors during device design, poorly written device operating and maintenance procedures, and inadequate or no training in device use. Nonetheless, as indicated by a study reported in Ref. 28, over 50% of the alleged failures of medical devices were due to operators, actions taken by involved patients, maintenance, and service.

Radiotherapy is also prone to human errors. More specifically, various case histories in the use of nuclear materials for patient therapy illustrate the existence of opportunities for human error. Many such incidents can be found in the annals of the US Nuclear Regulatory Commission (USNRC), which has the authority over radioactive materials including their use in the medical field.[22] Two cases reported in those annals are as follows:

- A patient was administered 50 millicuries of radioactive materials instead of 3 millicuries as prescribed by the doctor.
- A patient was administered 100 rad of radioactive materials to the brain accidentally.

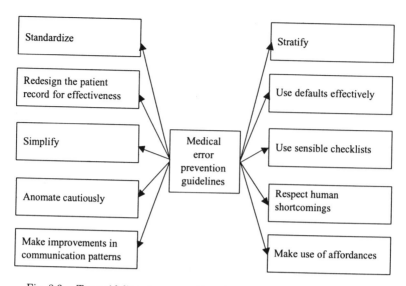

Fig. 8.3.   Ten guidelines for preventing the occurrence of medical errors.

8.6   General Guidelines for Preventing Medical Errors

Over the years various types of general guidelines have been developed to reduce the occurrence of medical errors.   Figure 8.3 presents ten such guidelines, namely: standardize, simplify, automate cautiously, make improvements in communication patterns, redesign the patient record, stratify, use defaults effectively, use sensible checklists, respect human short-comings, and make use of affordances.[29]

The guideline, standardize, is concerned with limiting the unnecessary variety in equipment, drugs, rules, and supplies. Past experiences indicate that when a procedure is repeated all the time, the probability of doing it incorrectly is reduced significantly. The guideline, simplify, calls for reducing the number of steps in a work process, the non-essential equipment, software, and procedures, as well as the number of times an instruction is given, and so on. All in all, simplicity leads to reduced chances for the occurrence of human errors.

The guideline, automate cautiously, basically warns us not to over-automate because over-automation may prevent operators or others from judging the true state of the system. Furthermore, it may create an illusion of safety, thus resulting in the decrease in human vigilance. The guideline, make improvements in communication patterns, calls for team members in operating rooms, intensive care units, and emergency departments to repeat orders to make sure that they have understood them correctly.

The guideline, redesign the patient record, is concerned with examining the effectiveness of the present form of records keeping and then taking appropriate measures. Remember that some patient record keeping could be too voluminous with buried important information. The guideline, stratify, basically warns against over-standardization (e.g. one size fits all) because it can cause errors.

The guideline, use defaults effectively, is concerned with making the correct action the easiest one. A default may simply be described as a standard order or a rule that works if nothing else intervenes. The guideline, use sensible checklists, calls for establishing and using checklists in a sensible and effective manner. Although checklists and procedures minimize variables and provide a greater possibility of consistent results, when they become something other than tools, they can certainly take away human judgment.

The guideline, respect human shortcomings, is concerned with considering factors such as stress, time pressure, memory limitations, workload, and circadian rhythm in designing tasks and work systems. Various types of errors may occur if factors such as these are not considered carefully during task and work systems' design. For example, people can easily forget to complete vital tasks under the environment of frequent interruptions. An example of rectification in a medical area could be, say, instead of having a physician to try to remember a dosage, a system should be designed where the information is presented to him/her on a computer or a checklist. The guideline, make use of affordances, is concerned with designing features in items that ensure correct use by providing clues to proper operation. For example, most automobiles with automatic transmissions would not start unless the gearshift is in the park position. All in all, it may be added that in the medical field it may not be possible to eradicate all errors, but their occurrence can be reduced.

8.7   Human Error Cost in Medical System

The occurrence of human error in the medical system not only leads to the unfortunate health consequences suffered by people, but also the high costs borne by society as a whole. Direct costs simply refer to higher health care related expenditures and the indirect costs include disability costs, personal costs of care, and lost productivity costs.

It is estimated that in the United States, the annual national cost of adverse events is around $38 billion and in turn, $17 billion of it is considered to be associated with preventable adverse events. Furthermore, for every dollar spent on drugs in nursing facilities, approximately one dollar and thirty cents are consumed in the treatment of drug-associated morbidity and mortality, translating into a total $7.6 billion for the entire nation. It is estimated that $3.6 billion of this amount is avoidable.[4,30]

8.7.1   *Health Care Human Error-Related Cost Studies*

Over the years various health care human error-related cost studies have been performed. Some of these studies are discussed below:

- **Thomas *et al. Study*.**[31] This study examined the medical records of 14732 randomly chosen discharges from 28 Colorado and Utah hospitals and a total of 459 adverse events were found, of which 265 were considered preventable. The total estimated cost of all these adverse events was $661889000, of which preventable adverse events accounted for $308382000.
- **Bloom Study.**[32] This study performed analysis of all direct costs associated with the care of 527 Medicaid recipients treated for arthritis with non-steroidal anti-inflammatory drugs (NSAIDS) for the period of December 1981 to November 1983. The study revealed that approximately $4 million was spent on treating preventable gastrointestinal adverse drug reactions to NSAIDS.
- **Bates *et al. Study*.**[5] This study examined 4108 admissions to a stratified random sample of 11 medical and surgical units in two hospitals over a period of six months (i.e. from February 1993 to July 1993). The study revealed that a total of 247 adverse drug events (ADEs) occurred among 207 admissions, of which 60 were preventable. The total annual costs incurred by a hospital due to both ADEs and preventable ADEs were $5.6 million and $2.8 million, respectively. Moreover, the study projected the national annual costs of all ADEs and preventable ADEs in the order of $4 billion and $2 billion, respectively.
- **Schneider *et al.*[33]** This study examined 109 patients at a hospital known to have had some clinical consequences from a medication error or adverse drug reaction (ADR). The study detected a total of 1911 adverse drug reactions and medical errors and estimated their annual cost to be around $1.5 million.

8.7.2 *Health Care Human Error Cost Estimation Models*

In the published literature, there are a large number of mathematical models available to estimate various types of costs.[34,35] Similarly, this section presents two mathematical models for estimating human error-related costs in health care.

Health Care Human Error Cost Estimation Model

The total cost of human error in health care is expressed by:

$$HCHETC = HEPC + HEOC, \tag{8.1}$$

where

HCHETC   is the health care human error total cost.

HEPC   is the human error prevention cost. This includes the cost of human error analysis, preventive measures, and information retrieval.

HEOC   is the human error occurrence cost. This includes the cost of damaged facilities, lost wages (if applicable), continuously following of the wrong path (if applicable), and liability suits.

Medical Device Human Error Cost Estimation Model

A medical device human error-related cost is expressed by:

$$TMDHEC = HEPC + IHEOC + EHEOC, \tag{8.2}$$

where

TMDHEC   is the total medical device human error cost.

HEPC   is the human error prevention cost. More specifically, this cost is associated with human error prevention activities at the device manufacturer's facilities.

IHEOC   is the internal human error occurrence cost. More specifically, this cost is associated with the device-related human error occurrence at the manufacturer's facilities (i.e. prior to the delivery of the device to the users).

EHEOC   is the external human error occurrence cost. More specifically, this cost is associated with the device-related human error occurrence after the delivery of the device to users.

Problems

1. Define the following terms:

   - Intensive care unit
   - Emergency medicine
   - Operating room

2. List at least five facts and figures concerned with human error in intensive care units.
3. What are the basic factors for the occurrence of human errors in intensive care units?
4. Write an essay on the occurrence of human errors in emergency medicine.
5. Write down at least five questions useful for reducing the occurrence of human errors in emergency medicine.
6. Write down the type of people that form a typical operating room team.
7. What are the main elements of the model of operating room performance?
8. Discuss the occurrence of human error in the following two areas:

   - Medical technology use
   - Image interpretation

9. List at least ten general guidelines for preventing the occurrence of medical errors.
10. Discuss at least two studies concerned with health care human error-related cost.

References

1. Classen, D.C., Pestotnik, S.L., Evans, R.S., *et al.*, "Computerized Surveillance of Adverse Drug Events in Hospital Patients," *Journal of the American Medical Association (JAMA)*, Vol. 266, 1991, pp. 2847–2851.
2. Wears, R.L. and Leape, L.L., "Human Error in Emergency Medicine," *Annals of Emergency Medicine*, Vol. 34, No. 3, 1999, pp. 370–372.
3. Mehta, R.H. and Eagle, K.A., "Missed Diagnoses of Acute Coronary Syndromes in the Emergency Rooms: Continuing Challenges," *The New England Journal of Medicine*, Vol. 342, No. 16, 2000, pp. 1207–1209.
4. Kohn, L.T., Corrigan, J.M., and Donaldson, M.S., (eds), *To Err Is Human: Building a Safer Health System*, Institute of Medicine, National Academy of Medicine, National Academy Press, Washington, D.C., 1999.

5. Bates, D.W., Spell, N.S., Cullen, D.J., *et al.*, "The Costs of Adverse Drug Events in Hospitalized Patients," *JAMA*, Vol. 277, No. 4, 1997, pp. 307–311.

6. Hospital Statistics: 1979 Edition, American Hospital Association, Chicago, 1979.

7. Knaus, W.A., Wagner, D.P., Draper, E.A., *et al.*, "The Range of Intensive Care Services Today," *JAMA*, Vol. 246, No. 23, 1981, pp. 2711–2716.

8. Wright, D., *Critical Incident Reporting in An Intensive Care Unit*, Report, Western General Hospital, Edinburgh, Scotland, UK, 1999.

9. Bracco, D., Favre, J.B., Bissonnette, B., *et al.*, "Human in a Multidisciplinary Intensive Care Unit: A 1-year Prospective Study," *Intensive Care Medicine*, Vol. 27, 2001, pp. 137–145.

10. Donchin, Y., Gopher, D., Olin, M., *et al.*, "A Look Into the Nature and Causes of Human Errors in the Intensive Care Unit," *Critical Care Medicine*, Vol. 23, No. 2, 1995, pp. 294–300.

11. Beckmann, V., Baldwin, I., Hart, G.K., *et al.*, "The Australian Incident Monitoring Study in Intensive Care (AIMS-ICU): An Analysis of the First Year of Reporting," *Anesthesia and Intensive Care*, Vol. 24, No. 3, 1996, pp. 320–329.

12. Abramson, N.S., Wald, K.S., Grenvik, A.N.A., *et al.*, "Adverse Occurrences in Intensive Care Units," *JAMA*, Vol. 244, No. 14, 1980, pp. 1582–1584.

13. Leape, L.L., Cullen, D.J., Clapp, M.D., *et al.*, "Pharmacist Participation on Physician Rounds and Adverse Drug Events in the Intensive Care Unit," *JAMA*, Vol. 282, No. 3, 1999, pp. 267–270.

14. Kyriacou, D.N. and Coben, J.H., "Errors in Emergency Medicine: Research Strategies," *Academic Emergency Medicine*, Vol. 7, No. 11, 2000, pp. 1201–1203.

15. Bogner, M.S., (ed), *Human Error in Medicine*, Lawrence Erlbaum Associates Publishers, Hillsdale, New Jersey, 1994.

16. Espinosa, J.A. and Nolan, T.W., "Reducing Errors Made by Emergency Physicians in Interpreting Radiographs: Longitudinal Study," *British Medical Journal*, Vol. 320, 2000, pp. 737–740.

17. Brady, W.J., Perron, A., and Ullman, E., "Errors in Emergency Physician Interpretation of ST-segment Elevation in Emergency Department Chest Pain Patients," *Academic Emergency Medicine*, Vol. 7, No. 11, 2000, pp. 1256–1260.

18. Pope, J.H., Aufderheide, T.P., Ruthazer, R., *et al.*, "Missed Diagnoses of Acute Cardiac Ischemia in the Emergency Department," *The New England Journal of Medicine*, Vol. 342, No. 16, 2000, pp. 1163–1170.

19. Rothman, K.J., Lanes, S., and Robins, J., "Casual Inference," *Epidemiology*, Vol. 4, 1993, pp. 555–556.

20. Robertson, L., *Injury Epidemiology: Research and Control Strategies*, Oxford University Press, New York, 1998.

21. Helmreich, R.L. and Schaefer, H.G., "Team Performance in the Operating Room, in Human Error in Medicine," M.S. Bogner, (ed), Lawrence Erlbaum Associates Publishers, Hillsdale, New Jersey, 1994, pp. 225–253.

22. VanCott, H., "Human Errors: Their Causes and Reduction," in *Human Error in Medicine*, M.S. Bogner, (ed), Lawrence Erlbaum Associates Publishers, Hillsdale, New Jersey, 1994, pp. 53–65.

23. Morrison, W.G. and Swann, I.J., "Electrocardiograph Interpretation by Junior Doctors," *Archives of Emergency Medicine*, Vol. 7, 1990, pp. 108–110.

24. Vincent, C.A., Driscoll, P.A., Audley, R.A., *et al.*, "Accuracy of Detection of Radiographic Abnormalities by Junior Doctors," *Archives of Emergency Medicine*, Vol. 5, 1988, pp. 101–109.

25. Rolland, J.P., Barrett, H.H., and Seeley, G.W., "Ideal Versus Human Observer for Long Tailed Point Spread Functions: Does De-convolution Help?" *Physiology, Medicine, and Biology*, Vol. 36, No. 8, pp. 1091–1109.

26. Squires, S., "Cholesterol Guessing Games," *Washington Post*, Washington, D.C., March 6, 1990.

27. Cooper, J.B., Newbower, R.S., and Kitz, R.J., "An Analysis of Major Errors and Equipment Failures in Anesthesia Management: Considerations for Prevention and Detection," *Anesthesiology*, Vol. 60, 1984, pp. 34–41.

28. Nobel, J.L., "Medical Device Failures and Adverse Effects," *Pediatric Emergency Care*, Vol. 7, 1991, pp. 120–123.

29. Crane, M., "How Good Doctors Can Avoid Bad Errors," *Medical Economics*, April 1997, pp. 36–43.

30. Bootman, J.L., Harrison, D., and Cox, E., "The Health Care Cost of Drug-Related Morbidity and Mortality in Nursing Facilities," *Archive of International Medicine*, Vol. 157, No. 18, 1997, pp. 2089–2096.

31. Thomas, E.J., Studdert, D.M., and Newhouse, J.P., "Costs of Medical Injuries in Utah and Colorado," *Inquiry*, Vol. 36, 1999, pp. 255–265.

32. Bloom, B.S., "Cost of Treating Arthritis and NSAID-Related Gastrointestinal Side-Effects," *Aliment. Pharmacol. Ther.*, Vol. 1, No. 2, 1998, pp. 131–138.

33. Schneider, P.J., Gift, M.G., Lee, Y.P., *et al.*, "Cost of Medication Related Problems at a University Hospital," *Am. J. Health-Syst. Pharm.*, Vol. 52, 1995, pp. 2415–2418.

34. Dhillon, B.S., *Life Cycle Costing: Techniques, Models, and Applications*, Gordon and Breach Science Publishers, New York, 1989.

35. Dhillon, B.S., *Medical Device Reliability and Associated Areas*, CRC Press, Boca Raton, Florida, 2000.

Chapter 9

Human Factors in Medical Devices

9.1 Introduction

Human factor problems are frequently encountered in medical devices and design-induced errors in that the use of such devices can result in patient injuries and deaths. The operating characteristics of the equipment can directly influence a user's behavior and misleading or illogical user interfaces can induce errors even by the most experienced users. More specifically, often-serious errors are committed by highly competent people, and poor device design is frequently sighted to be the significant causing factor.

Errors such as these usually cannot be eradicated simply by offering additional training or adding labels. The likelihood of user error increases significantly when a medical device is designed without giving proper attention to the cognitive, perceptual, and the physical abilities of the user. Often, stressful, noisy, and poorly lit operating environment coupled with poor device design increases the burden on the user. In addition, medical device human factors-related problems include poor training, poorly documented instructions, and limitations in the capabilities and experience of both professional and lay users.[1]

This chapter presents the various different aspects of human factors in medical devices.

9.2   Facts and Figures

Some of the facts and figures directly or indirectly concerned with human factors in medical devices are as follows:

- The Food and Drug Administration (FDA) in the US receives around 100000 reports through the medical device reporting (MDR) route and 5000 reports through the voluntary MedWatch program annually.[2] A significant number of these reports are concerned with human factor problems.
- Human errors cause or contribute to up to 90% of accidents in medical devices.[3-5]
- FDA's Center for Devices and Radiological Health (CDRH) reported that approximately 60% of the deaths or serious injuries associated with medical devices were due to user error.[6,7]
- During the period of January 1990–June 1995, the FDA received a total of 102 reports concerning head and body entrapment incidents involving hospital bedside rails. These incidents resulted in a number of deaths and injuries including a 2-year-old patient.[2]
- A study of the FDA incident reports on the Abbott Patient Controlled Analgesia (PCA) infuser revealed that approximately 68% of the fatalities and serious injuries were due to human error.[8]
- An amount of $375000 was paid out by a hospital in a settlement involving the death of a patient due to an infusion pump being erroneously set to deliver 210 cc of heparin per hour instead of the ordered 21 cc.[9]
- A fatal radiation-overdose accident was caused by a human error involving a Therac radiation therapy device.[10]
- The death of a patient receiving oxygen occurred when a concentrator pressure hose loosened and the intensity of alarm was not loud enough to be heard effectively over the drone of the device.[11]
- A patient died because of impeded airflow resulting from upside-down installation of an oxygen machine component.[11]
- Many patient deaths and injuries occurred because of the insertion of a cassette by users from one infusion pump model into another incompatible model.[11,12]
- During the time period of 1983–1991, a total of 2792 quality problems resulted in the recalls of medical devices and many of these problems were directly or indirectly related to human factors.[13]

9.3   Human Error Causing User-Interface Design Problems, Medical Devices with a High Incidence of Human Errors, and Medical Device-Associated Operator Errors

There are many user-interface device design problems that tend to "invite" the occurrence of a user error. Some of these problems are as follows[1]:

- Poor device design resulting in unnecessarily complex installation and maintenance tasks.
- Unconventional or complex arrangements of items such as displays, controls, and tubing.
- Poorly designed or inadequate labels.
- Difficult to remember, and/or rather confusing device operating instructions.
- Hard to read or ambiguous displays.
- Poor device feedback or status indication that result in user uncertainty.
- Unnecessarily intrusive or confusing device associated alarms.

Past experiences indicate that on the average errors in the use of medical devices result in at least three deaths or serious injuries per day.[14]

Over the years, various studies have been conducted to highlight medical devices with a high occurrence of human error. Table 9.1 presents the devices in the order of least error-prone to most error-prone.[6,14]

Past experiences indicate that there are numerous operator-associated errors that occur during the operation of medical devices or equipment. Some of these errors are as follows[15]:

- Misinterpretation of critical device outputs.
- Wrong decision making.
- Taking incorrect actions in critical situations.
- Mistakes in setting device/equipment parameters.
- Wrong improvization.
- Failure to recognize effectively the critical device outputs.
- Failure to follow prescribed instructions and procedures effectively.
- Inadvertent or untimely activation of controls.
- Wrong selection of devices/equipment with regard to clinical requirements and objectives.
- Over-reliance on automatic features, capabilities, or alarms of medical devices.

Table 9.1.   Medical devices with a high incidence of human error (i.e. in the order of least error-prone to most error-prone).

Order No.	Device Name
1 (least error-prone)	Continuous ventilators (respirators)
2	External low-energy defibrillator
3	Transluminal coronary angioplasty catheter
4	Catheter guide wire
5	Catheter introducer
6	Peritoneal dialysate delivery system
7	Implantable pacemaker
8	Mechanical/hydraulic impotence device
9	Non-powered suction apparatus
10	Electrosurgical cutting and coagulation device
11	Urological catheter
12	Infusion pump
13	Intra-vascular catheter
14	Implantable spinal cord simulator
15	Permanent pacemaker electrode
16	Administration kit for peritoneal dialysis
17	Orthodontic bracket aligner
18	Balloon catheter
19 (most error-prone)	Glucose meter

9.4   An Approach to Human Factors in the Development Process of Medical Devices for Reducing Human Errors, Areas for Questions in Developing an Effective Medical Device Design, and Characteristics of Well-Designed Medical Devices

Medical device or equipment designers are in a good position to recognize the potential for human errors and drastically reduce their occurrences.[11,16] The occurrence of human errors can be reduced quite significantly by considering human factors as an integral part of the medical device/equipment development process phases: concept phase, allocation of functions and preliminary design phase, pre-production prototype phase, market test and evaluation phase, final design phase, and production phase.[17]

During the concept phase, the human factors specialists perform tasks such as evaluating competitive devices, conducting analysis of industry and regulatory standards, interviewing potential users, working along with market researchers, and helping to develop and implement questionnaires. Also, these specialists evaluate proposed operations of potential devices with respect to various factors including educational background, skill range, and experiences of intended users in addition to the identification of device use environments. Some examples of the device use environments are: operating rooms critical care facilities, clinics and homes, emergency rooms, and patient units. Moreover, the medical device use is influenced by external environmental factors such as light, sound levels, and other devices in close proximity.[18]

In the allocation of functions and preliminary design phase, both the human factors and design professionals work together in determining which device functions should be automated and which will need manual points of interface between humans and the device. The manual points of interface may simply be described as operations in which humans have to monitor and control so that the required output/feedback from the medical device/equipment is obtained in an effective manner. The preliminary design is examined with respect to factors such as the operating environment of the device and the skills of the most untrained users. Generally, under normal circumstances, this task is executed by taking into consideration the reactions of potential device users and the drawings or sketches of the device operational environments.

During the pre-production prototype phase the device is evaluated and the prototype is built or updated after receiving additional evaluation and market test related information.

During the market test and evaluation phase the actual testing of the device is carried out and the feedback received from the market test is thoroughly examined by human factors, engineering, and marketing professionals.

In the final design phase, the design of the device is finalized by incorporating any human-factors-associated changes highlighted by the test, evaluation, and marketing phases.

During the production phase, the device is manufactured and then put on the market. Here the human factors professional monitors its performance and then performs the appropriate analysis of any proposed design changes, thereafter provides the appropriate assistance in the development of user-related training programs.

During the device design, there are many areas in which questions may be asked regarding simpler designs which are more intuitive and less demanding or more forgiving of user error. Some of those areas are as follows[18]:

- Displays and controls.
- User adjustments or manipulation requirements.
- Maintenance requirements.
- Difficulties with respect to maintenance/service.
- Device misassembly.
- Alarms' complexity and variation.
- Variables which the user has to interact with.
- Accuracy and speed of user interactions.
- Ability of alarms/feedback detecting errors/fault conditions.
- User training requirements.

Some of the characteristics of well-designed medical devices with respect to users are as follows[1]:

- Logical and confusion free.
- Consistent with the experiences of user community.
- Immediately alert users when device-related problems occur.
- Minimize the requirement for memory and performing mental calculations.
- Stop users from making fatal errors.
- Contain readable and comprehensible labels.
- Avoid overtaxing strength, visual capacity, dexterity, strength, or auditory capacity of users.

9.5   Rules of Thumb for Device Control/Display Arrangement and Design, Installation, Software Design, and Alarms with Respect to Users

Over the years, many rules of thumb have been developed to reduce directly or indirectly the occurrence of user error in medical devices. This section presents the rules of thumb for device control/display arrangement and design, installation, software design, and related alarms, separately.[11]

9.5.1 *Rules of Thumb for Device Control/Display Arrangement and Design to Avoid User Errors*

Some of these rules of thumb are as follows[11]:

- Ensure that workstations, displays, and controls are designed based on the user's basic capabilities (i.e. memory, hearing, vision, strength, reach, and dexterity).
- Ensure that the pitch and intensity of auditory signals are able to be heard effectively by the device user community.
- Ensure that all facets of device design are as consistent with user expectations as possible.
- Ensure that knobs, switches, and keys are designed and arranged in such a way that they minimize the likelihood of inadvertent activation.
- Ensure that the control and display arrangements are well-organized and uncluttered.
- Ensure that control knobs and switches are designed so that they correspond to the conventions of the user community.
- Ensure that all displays and labels are made so that they can be read effectively from typical viewing distances and angles.
- Ensure that all controls provide effective tactile feedback.
- Ensure the consistency of the abbreviations, symbols, text, and acronyms that are placed on the device by checking with the instructional manual.
- Ensure that effective brightness of visual signals can be perceived by the user community working under various illumination levels.
- Ensure that switches, control knobs, and keys are spaced sufficiently apart for easy manipulation.
- Ensure that color and shape coding are used as appropriate for facilitating the rapid identification of controls and displays.

9.5.2 *Rules of Thumb for Device Installation to Avoid User Errors*

Some of these rules of thumb are as follows[11]:

- Ensure that the user instructions are comprehensible and the warnings are conspicuous.
- Ensure that the components and accessories are properly numbered so that the defective ones can be effectively replaced with the good ones.

- Ensure that connectors, tubing, leuers, cables, and other hardware are properly designed for easy installation and connection.
- Ensure that textual complexity in maintenance documents is reduced considerably by adding in the appropriate graphics.
- Ensure that the positive locking mechanisms are present when there is a possibility of compromising the integrity of connections by factors such as component durability, motion, or casual contact.
- Avoid exposed electrical contacts as much as possible.

9.5.3   *Rules of Thumb for Device Software Design to Avoid User Errors*

Some of these rules of thumb are as follows[1]:

- Ensure that all users are kept up to date about the current device status.
- Avoid contradicting the expectations of users.
- Ensure that only design procedures that entail easy-to-remember steps are employed.
- Avoid confusing or overloading users with information that is densely packed, unformatted, or too brief.
- Avoid over using software in situations where a simple and straight forward hardware solution is feasible.
- Ensure that only the accepted symbols, colors, icons, and abbreviations are used for conveying information quickly, reliably, and economically.
- Ensure that only conspicuous mechanisms are provided for correction and troubleshooting guides.
- Ensure that dedicated displays or display sectors for critical information are considered seriously.
- Ensure that immediate and clear feedback is provided following user entries.
- Ensure that the design and use of symbols, headings, abbreviations, and formats are consistent and unambiguous.

9.5.4   *Rules of Thumb for Device Related Alarms*

Some of these rules of thumb are as follows[11]:

- Ensure that in designing and testing alarms, a wide spectrum of operating environments is considered.

- Ensure that alarms are designed so that they meet or exceed usual visual and hearing limitations of the typical user community.
- Ensure that only those codes that correspond to established conventions are used.
- Ensure that alarms are designed so that can easily be distinguished from one another, particularly from alarms on other medical devices in the same vicinity.
- Ensure that priority is given to critical alarms.
- Ensure that auditory and visual alerts and critical alarms are included in the medical device/equipment design requirements.
- Ensure that careful consideration is given to the effects of over-sensitivity, static electricity, and electromagnetic interference on alarm operation.
- Ensure that both color contrast and brightness contrast are effective under varying illumination conditions.

9.6 Evaluating Medical Devices Prior to Purchase and Already-Purchased with Respect to Human Factors and Practical General Guidelines for Alleviating Device-Interface Design Problems

Prior to procuring a medical device, it is essential to assess its usability; particularly, if it is to be used in life-sustaining or life-supporting areas. The following guidelines could be quite useful in this regard[11]:

- Ascertain if the manufacturer has performed adequate device human factors/usability testing.
- Consult other facilities/organizations that have already been using the device regarding their human factors-related experiences.
- Consult published evaluation results of the device under consideration.
- Negotiate a trial period prior to the actual procurement of the device under consideration.
- Consult the staff of other facilities concerning the predecessor device models produced by the same manufacturer.

In evaluating the medical devices procured, some indications of human-factor related problems are as follows[11]:

- Slow and arduous training.
- Frequent malfunctioning of alarms and batteries.
- Difficulty in hearing or distinguishing alarms.

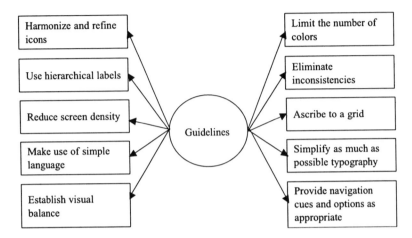

Fig. 9.1.   Practically inclined general guidelines for alleviating medical device interface design problems.

- Users complaining that the installation of accessories is confusing, difficult, or time-consuming.
- Tendency of staff/users to modify the device or take shortcuts.
- Only handfuls of staff members appear to be effectively using the device.
- Device components become detached frequently.
- Often, staff members refuse to use the device.
- Poorly labeled or located device controls.
- Difficulty in reading or understanding displays.
- Very annoying device alarms.
- Illogical and confusing device operations.
- Installation of wrong accessories.

Some of the practically inclined general guidelines for alleviating device-interface design problems are presented in Fig. 9.1.[19] Each of these guideline is discussed in detail in Refs. 6 and 19.

9.7   Human Error Analysis Methods for Medical Devices

Over the years many human error and safety analysis methods have been developed.[3,20–21] Some of these methods can be used to reduce directly or indirectly the occurrence of human error in medical devices, and they are discussed in the following subsections.[3,6,20]

9.7.1 *Failure Mode and Effects Analysis (FMEA)*

This method was developed in the early 1950s to analyze flight control systems and today, it is one of the most widely used techniques to analyze engineering systems during their design stages, from reliability and safety aspects.[22] FMEA may simply be described as a structured analysis of a device/item/function that helps to identify potential failure modes, their causes, and the effects of failures on system operation. When the criticality of the failures is evaluated and the failure modes are assigned priorities, the method is called failure mode, effects, and criticality analysis (FMECA). The main steps in performing the FMEA are shown in Fig. 9.2.

All in all, the FMEA is a bottom-up approach because analysts start with individual parts or components and then logically determine the effects of their failure on the entire system. The method is described in detail in Chapter 5 and a comprehensive list of references on the method is given in Ref. 23.

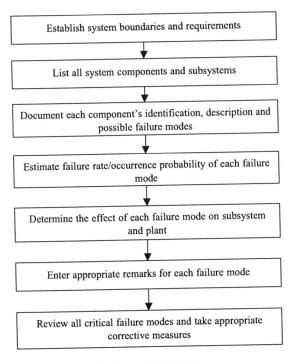

Fig. 9.2. FMEA Steps.

9.7.2   *Barrier Analysis*

This is based on the fact that a product has various types of energy that can result in property damage and injuries. Examples of such energy include mechanical impact, pharmaceutical reactions, and heat energy. This approach basically attempts to highlight the product/item associated energies and the suitable barriers for preventing these energies form reaching people or properties.[24]

Although the method appears to be somewhat abstract, it can be quite useful in identifying serious hazards quickly. In the event that an item has no designed-in barrier, the designers are alerted to incorporate one or more such barriers. A barrier could be physical, behavioral, or procedural. An example of a physical barrier is protective gloves which are used for protection against bloodbore pathogens. Examples of a behavior barrier include drug-interaction warnings because they influence the users' behavior.

9.7.3   *Fault Tree Analysis (FTA)*

This method was developed in the early 1960s in the Bell laboratories to analyze the Minuteman Launch Control System with regards to safety. Today the technique is widely used in the industrial sector to perform reliability and safety analysis of engineering systems and it can be used in performing human error analysis of medical devices.

FTA begins by first identifying an undesirable event of a system under consideration. This event is also called the top event of the system. Fault events that could cause the occurrence of top events are generated and connected by logic operators such as OR and AND. The OR gate provides a true output (fault) if one or more inputs (faults) are true and on the other hand, the AND gate provides a true output (fault) only if all the inputs (faults) are true.

The construction of a fault tree proceeds by the generation of events in a successive manner until the events (basic fault events) do not require to be developed any further. A fault tree is simply a logic structure relating the top events to the basic fault events.

The FTA method is described in detail in Chapter 5 and a comprehensive list of references on the technique is given in Ref. 25.

9.7.4   *Force Field Analysis (FFA)*

This method is often used in total quality management (TQM) studies and it can also be used in the human error analysis of medical devices.

The method calls for, first the identification of desirable outcomes of product usage and then the identification of forces that may push users toward and away from these outcomes. These forces could either be real (physical) or virtual such as time, stress, procedures, and professionalism.[24] Although the FFA is not a very quantitatively inclined approach, it is quite useful in stimulating analytical thinking.

9.7.5 *Throughput Ratio Method*

This method was originally developed by the United States Navy and it basically determines the operability of man-machine interfaces/stations.[20,26] A control panel could be a good example of the interfaces/stations. Operability may simply be described as the extent to which the man-machine station performance satisfies the station design expectations.

The term "throughput" basically means transmission because the ratio is defined in terms of responses/items per unit time emitted by the operator. Nonetheless, the throughput ratio is expressed by:

$$\theta = \left[\left(\frac{x}{y}\right) - \gamma\right](100), \tag{9.1}$$

where

θ is the man-machine operability or throughput ratio expressed in percentage.

γ is the correction factor (i.e. correction for error or out-of-tolerance output).

x is the total number of throughput items generated per unit time.

y is the total number of throughput items to be generated per unit time to satisfy design expectations.

The correction factor, γ, is defined by:

$$\gamma = A_1 A_2, \tag{9.2}$$

where

$$A_1 = \left(\frac{n}{N}\right)\left(\frac{x}{y}\right), \text{ and} \tag{9.3}$$

$$A_2 = A_1 P_{fe} P_{om}^2. \tag{9.4}$$

The symbols used in Eqs. 9.3 and 9.4 are defined below:

P_{fe} is the function failure probability because of an error,
P_{om} is the probability that the operator will miss the error,
N is the number of trials in which the control-display operation is conducted, and
n is the number of trials in which the control-display operation is conducted wrongly.

All in all, this ratio can be used to determine the device/equipment acceptability, to redesign the evaluated design with respect to human factors, to compare the operabilities of alternative designs, and to establish system/device feasibility.

Example 9.1   Assume that the following data are given:

$$P_{fe} = 0.65, \ P_{om} = 0.55, \ N = 20, \ n = 5, \ x = 4, \ \text{and} \ y = 8.$$

What is the value of the man-machine operability ratio?

By substituting the given values into Eqs. 9.2 to 9.4, we get:

$$\gamma = (0.125)(0.0246) = 0.0031,$$

$$A_1 = \left(\frac{5}{20}\right)\left(\frac{4}{8}\right) = 0.125, \ \text{and}$$

$$A_2 = (0.125)(0.65)(0.55)^2 = 0.0246.$$

By inserting the given and calculated values into Eq. 9.1, we get:

$$\theta = \left[\left(\frac{4}{8}\right) - 0.0031\right](100)$$

$$= 49.69\%.$$

It means that the value of the man-machine operability index is approximately 50%.

9.7.6   *Critical Incident Technique (CIT)*

This technique can be used to perform human error analysis of medical devices that have already been sold and used. The method requires asking the device users whether they have observed/experienced near-accidents or injuries related to the device under consideration. Critical incidents are very useful indicators that a device or its usage might be hazardous; thus requires careful attention.

The method is discussed in more detail in Ref. 24.

Problems

1. Write an essay on human factors in medical devices.
2. List at least seven facts and figures concerning human factors/errors in medical devices.
3. Discuss important user-interface device design problems.
4. List at least 15 medical devices with a high incidence of human error.
5. Describe an approach for taking into consideration human factors in the medical device development process.
6. List at least ten important areas for questions in developing an effective medical device design.
7. What are the important characteristics of well-designed medical devices with respect to human factors.
8. Discuss the rules of thumb for device control/display arrangement and design.
9. Discuss the guidelines for evaluating medical devices prior to procurement with respect to human factors.
10. Describe three important human error analysis methods useful for medical devices.

References

1. Rachlin, J.A., "Human Factors and Medical Devices," *FDA User Facility Reporting: A Quarterly Bulletin to Assist Hospitals, Nursing Homes, and Other Device User Facilities*, Issue No. 12, 1995, pp. 86–89.
2. "Improving Patient Care by Reporting Problems with Medical Devices," A *MedWatch Continuing Education Article, Food and Drug Administration (FDA)*, Rockville, Maryland, September 1997, pp. 1–8.
3. Maddox, M.E., "Designing Medical Devices to Minimize Human Error," *Medical Device Diagnostic Industry Magazine*, Vol. 19, No. 5, 1997, pp. 160–180.
4. Nobel, J.L., "Medical Device Failures and Adverse Effects," *Pediat. Emerg. Care*, Vol. 7, 1991, pp. 120–123.
5. Bogner, M.S., "Medical Devices and Human Error," in *Human Performance in Automated Systems: Current Research and Trends*, M. Mouloua and

R. Parasuraman (eds), Lawrence Erlbaum Associates Publishers, Hillsdale, New Jersey, 1994, pp. 64–67.

6. Dhillon, B.S., *Medical Device Reliability and Associated Areas*, CRC Press, Inc., Boca Raton, Florida, 2000.

7. Bogner, M.S., "Medical Devices: A New Frontier for Human Factors," *CSE-RIAC Gateway*, Vol. 4, No. 1, 1993, pp. 12–14.

8. Lin, L., "An Ergonomically Redesigned Analgesia Delivery Device Proves Safer and More Efficient," *Proceedings of the Human Factors and Ergonomics Society Annual Meeting*, 1998, pp. 346–350.

9. Brueley, M.E., "Ergonomics and Error: Who is Responsible?" *Proceedings of the First Symposium on Human Factors in Medical Devices*, 1989, pp. 6–10.

10. Casey, S., *Set Phasers on Stun: and Other True Tales of Design Technology and Human Error*, Aegean Inc., Santa Barbara, California, 1993.

11. Swayer, D., *Do it by Design: an Introduction to Human Factors in Medical Devices*, Center for Devices and Radiological Health, Food and Drug Administration, Washington, D.C., 1996.

12. Kortstra, J.R.A., "Designing for the User," *Medical Device Technology*, January/February, 1995, pp. 22–28.

13. Wallace, D.R. and Kuhn, D.R., *Lessons from 342 Medical Device Failures*, Information Technology Laboratory, National Institute of Standards and Technology, Gaithersburg, Maryland, 2000.

14. Wikland, M.E., *Medical Device and Equipment Design*, Interpharm Press, Inc., Buffalo Grove, Illinois, 1995.

15. Hyman, W.A., "Human Factors in Medical Devices," *Encyclopaedia of Medical Devices and Instrumentation*, J.G. Webster (ed), Vol. 3, John Wiley and Sons, New York, 1988, pp. 1542–1553.

16. ANSI/AAMI HE48, *Human Factors Engineering Guidelines and Preferred Practices for the Design of Medical Devices*, Association for the Advancement of Medical Instrumentation (AAMI), Arlington, Virginia, 1993.

17. Le Cocq, A.D., "Application of Human Factors Engineering in Medical Product Design," *Journal of Clinical Engineering*, Vol. 12, No. 4, 1987, pp. 271–277.

18. *Human Factors Points to Consider for Investigational Device Exemption (IDE) Devices*, a five page document, Office of Health and Industry Programs, Division of Device User Programs and Systems Analysis, Center for Devices and Radiological Health (CDRH), US Food and Drug Administration, Rockville, Maryland, 2001.

19. Wiklund, M.E., "Making Medical Device Interfaces More User-friendly," *Med. Dev. Diag. Ind. Mag.*, Vol. 20, No. 5, 1998, pp. 177–186.

20. Dhillon, B.S., *Human Reliability: With Human Factors*, Pergamon Press, Inc., New York, 1986.

21. "System Safety Analytical Techniques," *Safety Engineering Bulletin*, No. 3, May 1971, Available from the Electronic Industries Association, Washington, D.C.

22. Countinho, J.S., "Failure-effect Analysis," *Transactions of the New York Academy of Sciences*, Vol. 26, 1964, pp. 564–584.

23. Dhillon, B.S., "Failure Mode and Effect Analysis: Bibliography," *Microelectronics and Reliability*, Vol. 32, 1992, pp. 719–731.
24. Maddox, M.E., "Designing Medical Devices to Minimize Human Error," *Medical Device and Diagnostic Industry Magazine*, Vol. 19, No. 5, 1997, pp. 166–180.
25. Dhillon, B.S., *Reliability and Quality Control: Bibliography on General and Specialized Areas*, Beta Publishers, Inc., Gloucester, Ontario, 1992.
26. Meister, D., *Comparative Analysis of Human Reliability Models*, Report No. AD 734432, 1971, Available from the National Technical Information Service, Springfield, Virginia.

Chapter 10

Mathematical Models for Predicting Human Reliability and Error in Medical System

10.1 Introduction

In mathematical modeling, the components of an item are denoted by idealized elements having all the representative characteristics of real life components and whose behavior may be described by equations. The degree of realism of a mathematical model is subjected to the assumptions imposed upon it.

In scientific fields, mathematical models are widely used to study various types of physical phenomena. In particular over the years a large number of mathematical models have been developed to study human reliability and human error in scientific systems. Many of these models were developed by using stochastic processes including that presented by Markov.[1] Although, the usefulness of these models may vary from one situation to another, some of the human reliability and error models are successfully being used to represent various types of real life environments. Thus, some of these models can also be used to tackle human reliability and error-related problems in the health care system.

This chapter presents the mathematical models considered useful for predicting human reliability and error in the medical system.

10.2 Model I: Human Performance Reliability

Health care professionals may perform various types of tasks including time continuous tasks such as operating, monitoring, and tracking. A good

153

knowledge about the performance of these tasks successfully plays an important role in various key decisions. An expression for predicting the reliability
of performing such tasks may be developed as follows[2-4]:

The probability of error occurrence, say, in a health care task, in the
finite time interval Δt with event B given, is:

$$P(A/B) = \theta(t)\Delta t, \tag{10.1}$$

where

$\theta(t)$ is the time t dependent human error rate.
A is an event that human error will occur in the
time interval $[t, t + \Delta t]$.
B is an errorless performance event of duration t.

Thus the joint probability of the errorless performance is given by:

$$P(\bar{A}/B)P(B) = P(B) - P(A/B)P(B), \tag{10.2}$$

where

$P(B)$ is the probability of occurrence of event B.
$\bar{A}$ is the event that error will not occur in interval $[t, t + \Delta t]$.

It is to be noted that Eq. 10.2 represents an errorless performance probability over time intervals $[0, t]$ and $[t, t + \Delta t]$.

Equation 10.2 may be rewritten in the following form:

$$HR(t) - HR(t)P(A/B) = HR(t + \Delta t), \tag{10.3}$$

where $HR(t)$ is the human reliability at time t.

By inserting Eq. 10.1 into Eq. 10.3 and rearranging, we get:

$$\frac{HR(t + \Delta t) - HR(t)}{\Delta t} = -HR(t)\theta(t). \tag{10.4}$$

In the limiting case, Eq. 10.4 becomes

$$\lim_{\Delta t \to 0} \frac{HR(t + \Delta t) - HR(t)}{\Delta t} = \frac{dHR(t)}{dt} = -HR(t)\theta(t). \tag{10.5}$$

At time $t = 0$, $HR(t) = 0$.

By rearranging Eq. 10.5, we get:

$$\frac{1}{HR(t)} dHR(t) = -\theta(t)\, dt. \tag{10.6}$$

Integrating both sides of Eq. 10.6 over the time interval $[0,\ t]$, we write:

$$\int_1^{HR(t)} \frac{1}{HR(t)} \cdot dHR(t) = -\int_0^t \theta(t)\, dt. \tag{10.7}$$

After evaluating Eq. 10.7, we get

$$HR(t) = e^{-\int_0^t \theta(t)\, dt}. \tag{10.8}$$

The above expression can be used to compute human reliability for any time to human error statistical distribution (e.g. the Weibull, exponential, or Rayleigh distributions).

By integrating Eq. 10.8 over the time interval $[0,\ \infty]$ we get the following general expression for the mean time to human error (MTTHE)[1]:

$$MTTHE = \int_0^\infty e^{-\int_0^t \theta(t)\, dt}\, dt. \tag{10.9}$$

Example 10.1   Assume that a health care professional is performing a certain task and his/her times to human error are Weibull distributed. Thus the professional's time-dependent human error rate is defined by:

$$\theta(t) = \frac{\alpha t^{\alpha-1}}{\beta^\alpha}, \tag{10.10}$$

where

α is the Weibull shape parameter,
β is the Weibull scale parameter, and
t is time.

Obtain the following:

- Expressions for the professional's reliability and MTTHE.
- The professional's reliability for a 10-hour mission when $\alpha = 1$ and $\beta = 500$-hours (the health care professional's mean time to human error).

By substituting Eq. 10.10 into Eq. 10.8, we get:

$$\text{HR}(t) = e^{-\int_0^t ((\alpha t^{\alpha-1})/\beta^\alpha)\, dt}$$

$$= e^{-(t/\beta)^\alpha}. \tag{10.11}$$

Similarly, by inserting Eq. 10.11 into Eq. 10.9, we get:

$$\text{MTTHE} = \int_0^\infty e^{-(t/\beta)^\alpha}\, dt$$

$$= \beta\Gamma\left(1 + \frac{1}{\alpha}\right), \tag{10.12}$$

where

$\Gamma(\bullet)$ is the gamma function and is defined by:

$$\Gamma(y) = \int_0^\infty t^{y-1} e^{-t}\, dt, \quad \text{for } y > 0. \tag{10.13}$$

By substituting the specified data values into Eq. 10.11, we obtain:

$$\text{HR}(10) = e^{-(10/500)^1}$$

$$= 0.9802.$$

Expressions for the professional's reliability and MTTHE are given by Eqs. 10.11 and 10.12, respectively. The health care professional's reliability for the specified data values is approximately 98%.

10.3   Model II: Human Correctability Function

The human correctability function, $\text{CH}(t)$, is concerned with the correction of self-generated human errors and it may simply be described as the probability that a task error will be corrected in time t subjected to stress inherent in the nature of the task and its associated environments. Mathematically, the correctability function may be expressed as follows[2-4]:

$$\text{CH}(t) = P(\text{correction of human error in time } t/\text{stress}), \tag{10.14}$$

where P is the probability.

   The time derivative of not-correctability function, $\overline{\text{CH}}(t)$, may be defined as follows:

$$\overline{\text{CH}}'(t) = -\frac{1}{M} M_{\overline{C}}'(t), \tag{10.15}$$

where

The prime denotes differentiation with respect to time t,

$M_{\bar{C}}(t)$ is the number of times the task is not accomplished after time t, and

M is the number of times task correction is accomplished after time t.

Dividing the both sides of Eq. 10.15 by $M_{\bar{C}}(t)$ and rearranging, we get:

$$\frac{\overline{CH}'(t)M}{M_{\bar{C}}(t)} = \frac{M'_{\bar{C}}(t)}{M_{\bar{C}}(t)}. \qquad (10.16)$$

The right-hand side of Eq. 10.16 represents the instantaneous task correction rate $CR(t)$. Hence using Eq. 10.14 we write Eq. 10.16 in the following form:

$$\frac{\overline{CH}'(t)}{\overline{CH}(t)} + CR(t) = 0. \qquad (10.17)$$

By solving Eq. 10.17 for given initial conditions we get:

$$\overline{CH}(t) = e^{-\int_0^t CR(t)\,dt}. \qquad (10.18)$$

By using the relationship $\overline{CH}(t) + CH(t) = 1$ and Eq. 10.18 we get:

$$CH(t) = 1 - e^{-\int_0^t CR(t)\,dt}. \qquad (10.19)$$

Example 10.2   A health care professional is performing a certain task and his/her error correction times are Weibull distributed. Thus the professional's time dependent error or task correction rate is defined by:

$$CR(t) = \frac{bt^{b-1}}{\beta^b}, \qquad (10.20)$$

where

t is time,

b is the Weibull shape parameter, and

β is the Weibull scale parameter.

Obtain an expression for the professional's correctability function.

By substituting Eq. 10.20 into Eq. 10.19 we get:

$$CH(t) = 1 - e^{-\int_0^t ((bt^{b-1})/\beta^b)\, dt}$$

$$= 1 - e^{-(t/\beta)^b}. \tag{10.21}$$

The above equation is the expression for the professional's correctability function.

10.4   Model III: Human Performance Reliability in Alternating Environment

This model represents a health care professional performing time-continuous task under fluctuating environments (i.e. normal and stressful). Under this scenario the occurrence of human errors may vary quite significantly from normal environment to stressful environment. This model can be used to calculate the professional's performance reliability and his/her mean time to human error under the stated conditions.

The model state space diagram is shown in Fig. 10.1. The numerals in the boxes denote the health care professional's states. The other symbols used in the diagram are defined subsequently. The following assumptions are associated with this model[5]:

- Human error rates are constant.
- The rate of changing the health care professional's condition from normal to the stressful state and vice versa is constant.
- All human errors occur independently.

The following symbols were used to develop equations for the model:

i is the ith state of the health care professional; $i = 0$ means that the health care professional performs his/her task correctly in a normal environment, $i = 1$ means that the health care professional performs his/her task correctly in a stressful environment, $i = 2$ means that the health care professional has committed an error in a normal environment, $i = 3$ means that the health care professional has committed an error in a stressful environment.

$P_i(t)$ is the probability of the health care professional being in state i at time t, for $i = 0, 1, 2, 3$.

θ_n is the constant error rate of the health care professional under normal environment.

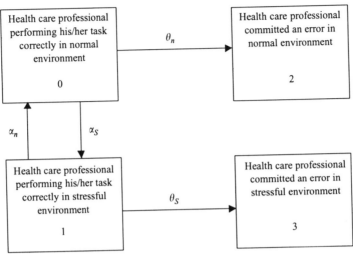

Fig. 10.1.   State space diagram for the health care professional working in normal and stressful environment.

θ_S is the constant error rate of the health care professional under stressful environment.

α_n is the constant transition rate from stressful environment to normal environment.

α_S is the constant transition rate from normal environment to stressful environment.

With the aid of the Markov method, we write down the following equations for Fig. 10.1[5]:

$$\frac{dP_0(t)}{dt} + (\theta_n + \alpha_S)P_0(t) = P_1(t)\alpha_n, \qquad (10.22)$$

$$\frac{dP_1(t)}{dt} + (\theta_S + \alpha_n)P_1(t) = P_0(t)\alpha_S, \qquad (10.23)$$

$$\frac{dP_2(t)}{dt} = P_0(t)\theta_n, \qquad (10.24)$$

$$\frac{dP_3(t)}{dt} = P_1(t)\theta_S. \qquad (10.25)$$

At time $t = 0$, $P_0(0) = 1$, and $P_1(0) = P_2(0) = P_3(0) = 0$.

By solving Eqs. 10.22–10.25 with the aid of the Laplace transforms, we get the following expressions for the state probabilities:

$$P_0(t) = (w_2 - w_1)^{-1}[(w_2 + \theta_s + \alpha_n)e^{w_2 t} - (w_1 + \theta_s + \alpha_n)e^{w_1 t}], \quad (10.26)$$

where

$$w_1 = [-a_1 + \sqrt{a_1^2 - 4a_2}]/2, \qquad (10.27)$$

$$w_2 = [-a_1 - \sqrt{a_1^2 - 4a_2}]/2, \qquad (10.28)$$

$$a_1 = \theta_n + \theta_S + \alpha_n + \alpha_S, \qquad (10.29)$$

$$a_2 = \theta_n(\theta_S + \alpha_n) + \alpha_S\theta_S, \qquad (10.30)$$

$$P_2(t) = a_4 + a_5 e^{w_2 t} - a_6 e^{w_1 t}, \qquad (10.31)$$

where

$$a_3 = \frac{1}{w_2 - w_1}, \qquad (10.32)$$

$$a_4 = \theta_n(\theta_S + \alpha_n)/w_1 w_2, \qquad (10.33)$$

$$a_5 = a_3(\theta_n + a_4 w_1), \qquad (10.34)$$

$$a_6 = a_3(\theta_n + a_4 w_2), \qquad (10.35)$$

$$P_1(t) = \alpha_s a_3(e^{w_2 t} - e^{w_1 t}), \qquad (10.36)$$

$$P_3(t) = a_7[(1 + a_3)(w_1 e^{w_2 t} - w_2 e^{w_1 t})], \qquad (10.37)$$

where

$$a_7 = \theta_S \alpha_S/w_1 w_2. \qquad (10.38)$$

The reliability of the health care professional is given by:

$$R_h(t) = P_0(t) + P_1(t), \qquad (10.39)$$

where $R_h(t)$ is the health care professional's reliability at time t.

By integrating Eq. 10.39 over the time interval $[0, \infty]$, we get the following expression for the health professional's mean time to human error:

$$\text{MTTHE}_h = \int_0^\infty R_h(t)\, dt$$

$$= (\theta_S + \alpha_S + \alpha_n)/a_2, \qquad (10.40)$$

where MTTHE_h is the health care professional's mean time to human error.

Example 10.3   Assume that a health care professional's error rates in normal and stressful environments are 0.003 errors/hour and 0.005 errors/hour, respectively. The transition rates from normal to stressful environment and vice-versa are 0.03 times per hour and 0.008 times per hour, respectively. Calculate the health care professional's mean time to human error.

By substituting the given data into Eq. 10.40, we get:

$$\text{MTTHE}_h = \frac{0.005 + 0.03 + 0.008}{0.003(0.005 + 0.008) + (0.03)(0.005)}$$

$$= 227.51 \text{ hours.}$$

Thus the health care professional's mean time to human error is 227.51 hours.

10.5   Model IV: Human Performance Reliability with Critical and Non-Critical Errors

This model represents a health care professional performing a time continuous task subjected to two types of errors: critical and non-critical. More specifically, the errors made by the professional are separated into two distinct categories, i.e. critical and non-critical. The model can be used to calculate the health care professional's performance reliability, the probability of him/her committing a critical human error, the probability of him committing a non-critical human error, and his/her mean time to human error.

The model state space diagram is shown in Fig. 10.2. The numerals in the boxes denote the health care professional's states. The other symbols used in the diagram are defined subsequently.

The model is subjected to the following assumptions:

- All human errors occur independently.
- Critical and non-critical error rates are constant.

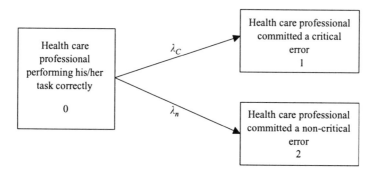

Fig. 10.2.   State space diagram for the health care professional subjected to critical and non-critical errors.

The following symbols are associated with the model:

i is the ith state of the health care professional; $i = 0$ means that the health care professional performing his/her task correctly, $i = 1$ means that the health care professional has committed a critical error, $i = 2$ means that the health care professional has committed a non-critical error.

λ_C is the constant critical error rate of the health care professional.

λ_n is the constant non-critical error rate of the health care professional.

$P_i(t)$ is the probability of the health care professional in state i at time t, for $i = 0, 1, 2$.

Using the Markov method, we write down the following equations for Fig. 10.2[6]:

$$\frac{dP_0(t)}{dt} + (\lambda_C + \lambda_n)P_0(t) = 0, \tag{10.41}$$

$$\frac{dP_1(t)}{dt} - \lambda_C P_0(t) = 0, \tag{10.42}$$

$$\frac{dP_2(t)}{dt} - \lambda_n P_0(t) = 0. \tag{10.43}$$

At time $t = 0$, $P_0(0) = 1$, $P_1(0) = 0$, and $P_2(0) = 0$.

By solving Eqs. 10.41–10.43, we get the following expressions for the health care professional's state probabilities[6]:

$$P_0(t) = e^{-(\lambda_C + \lambda_n)t}, \tag{10.44}$$

$$P_1(t) = \frac{\lambda_C}{\lambda_C + \lambda_n}[1 - e^{-(\lambda_C + \lambda_n)t}], \tag{10.45}$$

$$P_2(t) = \frac{\lambda_n}{\lambda_C + \lambda_n}[1 - e^{-(\lambda_C + \lambda_n)t}]. \tag{10.46}$$

Thus the health care professional's performance reliability is given by:

$$R_h(t) = P_0(t)$$
$$= e^{-(\lambda_C + \lambda_n)t}, \tag{10.47}$$

where $R_h(t)$ is the health care professional's performance reliability at time t.

By integrating Eq. 10.47 over the time interval $[0, \infty]$, we get the following expression for the health care professional's mean time to human error:

$$\text{MTTHE}_h = \int_0^\infty e^{-(\lambda_C + \lambda_n)t} dt$$

$$= \frac{1}{\lambda_C + \lambda_n}, \qquad (10.48)$$

where MTTHE_h is the health care professional's mean time to human error.

Example 10.4   Assume that a professional is performing a certain time continuous medical task and his/her constant critical and non-critical error rates are 0.002 errors/hour and 0.009 errors/hour, respectively. Calculate the professional's reliability, the probability of him/her committing a critical error, and probability of him/her committing a non-critical error during a 10-hour mission.

By substituting the given data values into Eqs. 10.44–10.46, we obtain:

$$P_0(10) = e^{-(0.002+0.009)(10)}$$

$$= 0.8958,$$

$$P_1(10) = \frac{0.002}{(0.002 + 0.009)}[1 - e^{(0.002+0.009)(10)}]$$

$$= 0.0189,$$

$$P_2(10) = \frac{0.009}{(0.002 + 0.009)}[1 - e^{(0.002+0.009)(10)}]$$

$$= 0.0852.$$

Thus the professional's reliability, the probability of him/her committing a critical error, and the probability of him/her committing a non-critical error are 0.8958, 0.0189, and 0.0852, respectively.

10.6   Model V: Human Performance Reliability with Critical and Non-Critical Errors and Corrective Action

This model is the same as Model IV but with one exception, i.e. the corrective action is considered by the health care professional from states 1 and 2 as shown in Fig. 10.3.[6] Symbols μ_C and μ_n are the health care professional's constant critical error correction rate and constant non-critical

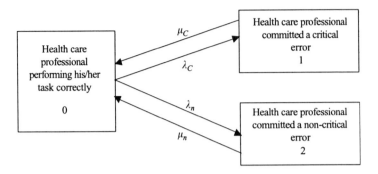

Fig. 10.3.   State space diagram for the health care professional subjected to critical and non-critical errors and corrections.

error correction rate, respectively. All other symbols and assumptions used in the model are identical to the ones in Model IV.

By using the Markov method, we write down the following equations for Fig. 10.3[6]:

$$\frac{dP_0(t)}{dt} + (\lambda_C + \lambda_n)P_0(t) = \mu_C P_1(t) + \mu_n P_2(t), \tag{10.49}$$

$$\frac{dP_1(t)}{dt} + \mu_C P_1(t) = \lambda_C P_0(t), \tag{10.50}$$

$$\frac{dP_2(t)}{dt} + \mu_n P_2(t) = \lambda_n P_0(t). \tag{10.51}$$

At time $t = 0$, $P_0(0) = 1$, and $P_1(0) = P_2(0) = 0$.

After solving Eqs. 10.49–10.51, we get the following state probability equations:

$$P_0(t) = \frac{\mu_C \mu_n}{m_1 m_2} + \left[\frac{(m_1 + \mu_n)(m_1 + \mu_C)}{m_1(m_1 - m_2)} \right] e^{m_1 t} - \left[\frac{(m_2 + \mu_n)(m_2 + \mu_C)}{m_2(m_1 - m_2)} \right] e^{m_2 t}, \tag{10.52}$$

where

$$m_1, m_2 = \frac{-a \pm \sqrt{a^2 - 4(\mu_C \mu_n + \lambda_C \mu_n + \lambda_n \mu_C)}}{2}, \tag{10.53}$$

$$a = \lambda_C + \lambda_n + \mu_C + \mu_n, \tag{10.54}$$

$$m_1 m_2 = \mu_C \mu_n + \lambda_n \mu_C + \lambda_C \mu_n, \tag{10.55}$$

$$m_1 + m_2 = -(\mu_C + \mu_n + \lambda_C + \mu_n), \tag{10.56}$$

$$P_1(t) = \frac{\lambda_C \mu_n}{m_1 m_2} + \left[\frac{\lambda_C m_1 + \lambda_C \mu_n}{m_1(m_1 - m_2)}\right] e^{m_1 t} - \left[\frac{(\mu_n + m_2)\lambda_C}{m_2(m_1 - m_2)}\right] e^{m_2 t}, \quad (10.57)$$

$$P_2(t) = \frac{\lambda_n \mu_C}{m_1 m_2} + \left[\frac{\lambda_n m_1 + \lambda_n \mu_C}{m_1(m_1 - m_2)}\right] e^{m_1 t} - \left[\frac{(\mu_C + m_2)\lambda_n}{m_2(m_1 - m_2)}\right] e^{m_2 t}. \quad (10.58)$$

Thus the health care professional's performance reliability with correction is given by Eq. 10.52, i.e.

$$R_{hC}(t) = P_0(t), \qquad (10.59)$$

where $R_{hC}(t)$ is the health care professional's performance reliability with correction at time t.

As time t becomes very large, we get the following steady state probabilities from Eqs. 10.52, 10.57, and 10.58, respectively:

$$P_0 = \lim_{t \to \infty} P_0(t) = \frac{\mu_C \mu_n}{m_1 m_2}, \qquad (10.60)$$

$$P_1 = \lim_{t \to \infty} P_1(t) = \frac{\lambda_C \mu_n}{m_1 m_2}, \qquad (10.61)$$

$$P_2 = \lim_{t \to \infty} P_2(t) = \frac{\lambda_n \mu_C}{m_1 m_2}, \qquad (10.62)$$

where P_i is the health care professional's steady state probability in state i; for $i = 0, 1, 2$.

Example 10.5 Assume that a health care professional is performing a time continuous task and during an accumulated period of 10000 hours he/she made five critical human errors and self-corrected two of them. During the same period, the professional also made ten non-critical human errors and self-corrected four of them. More specifically, he/she took two hours to correct both the critical errors and three hours to correct the four non-critical errors.

Calculate the health care professional's steady state probability of being in state 0, if the times to error and the times to error correction are exponentially distributed.

For the specified data values, we obtain

$$\lambda_C = \frac{5}{10000} = 0.0005 \text{ errors/hour},$$

$$\lambda_n = \frac{10}{10000} = 0.0001 \text{ errors/hour},$$

$$\mu_C = \frac{2}{2} = 1 \text{ correction/hour},$$

$$\mu_n = \frac{3}{4} = 0.75 \text{ corrections/hour}.$$

By substituting the above calculated values into Eq. 10.60, we get:

$$P_0 = \frac{(1)(0.75)}{(1)(0.75) + (0.001)(1) + (0.0005)(0.75)}$$

$$= 0.9982.$$

Thus the steady state probability of the health care professional being in state 0 is 0.9982.

10.7   Model VI: Reliability Analysis of a Medical Redundant System with Human Errors

This model represents a twin redundant active unit medical system subjected to human error. Each unit can fail either due to a hardware failure or a human error. At least one unit must operate normally for system success. The system state space diagram is shown in Fig. 10.4. The numerals in the circles, boxes, and diamond denote system states.

The model is subjected to the following assumptions[7]:

• Both the units operate simultaneously.
• Each unit can fail either due to a hardware failure or a human error.
• Hardware failure and human error rates are constant.
• Hardware failures and human errors occur independently.
• Both the units are identical.
• Each unit's failures can be grouped under two categories: failures due to hardware and failures due to human error.

The following symbols are associated with this model:

i is the ith state of the medical system; $i = 0$ means that both the units of the medical system working normally, $i = 1$ means that one

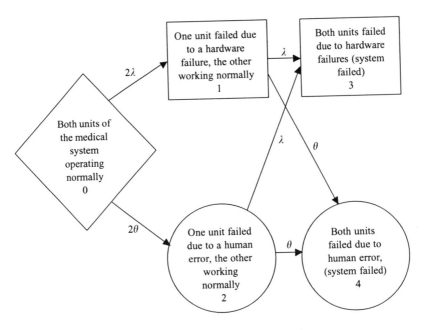

Fig. 10.4.   State space diagram of a two redundant unit medical system.

unit has failed due to a hardware failure, but the other is working normally, $i = 2$ means that one unit has failed due to a human error, but the other is working normally, $i = 3$ means that both the units have failed due to hardware failures, $i = 4$ means that both the units have failed due to human errors.

$P_i(t)$ is the probability that the medical system is in state i at time t, for $i = 0, 1, 2, 3, 4$.

λ is the constant hardware failure rate of a unit.

θ is the constant human error rate of a unit.

Using the Markov method, we write down the following equations for Fig. 10.4[1]:

$$\frac{dP_0(t)}{dt} + (2\lambda + 2\theta)P_0(t) = 0, \tag{10.63}$$

$$\frac{dP_1(t)}{dt} + (\lambda + \theta)P_1(t) = 2\lambda P_0(t), \tag{10.64}$$

$$\frac{dP_2(t)}{dt} + (\lambda + \theta)P_2(t) = 2\theta P_0(t), \tag{10.65}$$

$$\frac{dP_3(t)}{dt} = \lambda P_1(t) + \lambda P_2(t), \tag{10.66}$$

$$\frac{dP_4(t)}{dt} = \theta P_1(t) + \theta P_2(t). \tag{10.67}$$

At time $t = 0$, $P_0(0) = 1$, and $P_1(0) = P_2(0) = P_3(0) = P_4(0) = 0$.

By solving Eqs. 10.63–10.67, we get the following equations for the system state probabilities:

$$P_0(t) = e^{-2(\lambda+\theta)t}, \tag{10.68}$$

$$P_1(t) = \frac{2\lambda}{(\lambda+\theta)}[e^{-(\lambda+\theta)t} - e^{-2(\lambda+\theta)t}], \tag{10.69}$$

$$P_2(t) = \frac{2\theta}{(\lambda+\theta)}[e^{-(\lambda+\theta)t} - e^{-2(\lambda+\theta)t}], \tag{10.70}$$

$$P_3(t) = \frac{\lambda}{(\lambda+\theta)}[1 - e^{-(\lambda+\theta)t}]^2, \tag{10.71}$$

$$P_4(t) = \frac{\theta}{(\lambda+\theta)}[1 - e^{-(\lambda+\theta)t}]^2. \tag{10.72}$$

The medical system reliability is given by:

$$R_m(t) = P_0(t) + P_1(t) + P_2(t)$$
$$= 1 - [1 - e^{-(\lambda+\theta)t}]^2, \tag{10.73}$$

where $R_m(t)$ is the reliability of the medical system with human error.

By integrating Eq. 10.74 over the time interval $[0, \infty]$, we get:

$$\text{MTTF}_S = \int_0^\infty R_m(t)\, dt$$
$$= \frac{3}{2(\lambda+\theta)}, \tag{10.74}$$

where MTTF_S is the mean time to failure of a twin redundant unit medical system with human error.

Example 10.6   A medical system is composed of two independent, active, and identical units. At least one unit must operate normally for system success. Each unit can fail either due to a hardware failure or a human error. Each unit's constant hardware failure and human error rates are 0.006 failures/hour and 0.0005 errors/hour, respectively.

Calculate the system reliability for a 100-hour mission and the mean time to failure.

Using the specified data values in Eq. 10.73 we get:

$$R_m(100) = 1 - [1 - e^{-(0.006+0.0005)(100)}]^2$$
$$= 0.7716.$$

Similarly by using the given data values in Eq. 10.74 we get:

$$\text{MTTFs} = \frac{3}{2(0.006 + 0.0005)}$$
$$= 230.77 \text{ hours.}$$

Thus the medical system reliability and the mean time to failure are 0.7716 and 230.77 hours, respectively.

Problems

1. A health care professional is performing a certain task and his/her times to human error are Rayleigh distributed. Obtain an expression for the professional's reliability.

2. Assume that a professional is performing a certain medical-related task and his/her times to human error are exponentially distributed. Obtain an expression for the professional's mean time to human error.

3. Assume that in the above problem (i.e. Problem No. 2), the professional's mean time to human error is 500-hours. Calculate the professional's reliability for an 8-hour mission.

4. Prove that a health care professional's reliability is given by Eq. 10.8.

5. Define human correctability function.

6. For the specified data values in Example 10.3, calculate the health care professional's reliability for a 5-hour mission.

7. For the specified data values in Example 10.4, calculate the health care professional's mean time to human error.

8. Prove that in Model V, $P_0(t) + P_1(t) + P_2(t) = 1$.

9. Develop a state space diagram for Model VI by assuming that the redundant units are non-identical.

10. A medical system is composed of two independent, active, and identical units. At least one unit must operate normally for system success. Each unit can fail either due to a hardware failure or a human error. Each unit's constant hardware failure and human error rates are 0.004 failures/hour and 0.0006 errors/hour, respectively. Calculate the system reliability for a 50-hour mission and the mean time to failure.

References

1. Dhillon, B.S., *Human Reliability with Human Factors*, Pergamon Press, Inc., New York, 1986.
2. Regulinski, T.L. and Askren, W.B., "Mathematical Modeling of Human Performance Reliability," *Proceedings of the Annual Symposium on Reliability*, 1969, pp. 5–11.
3. Regulinski, T.L. and Askren, W.B., "Stochastic Modeling of Human Performance Effectiveness Functions," *Proceedings of the Annual Reliability and Maintainability Symposium*, 1972, pp. 407–416.
4. Askren, W.B. and Regulinski, T.L., "Quantifying Human Performance for Reliability Analysis of Systems," *Human Factors*, Vol. 11, 1969, pp. 393–396.
5. Dhillon, B.S., "Stochastic Models for Predicting Human Reliability," *Microelectronics and Reliability*, Vol. 25, 1985, pp. 729–752.
6. Dhillon, B.S., *Design Reliability: Fundamentals and Applications*, CRC Press, Inc., Boca Raton, Florida, 1999.
7. Dhillon, B.S. and Rayapati, S.N., "Reliability Analysis of Non-maintained Parallel Systems Subject to Hardware Failure and Human Error," *Microelectronics and Reliability*, Vol. 25, 1985, pp. 111–122.

Chapter 11

Health Care Human Error Reporting Systems and Data

11.1 Introduction

Human error data plays a key role in decisions concerning human error in health care system. The effectiveness of these decisions depends on the quality of error data (i.e. poor quality data will lead to ineffective decisions). It means to devote as much attention as possible when collecting and analyzing such data.

Currently, there are many human error-related reporting systems in use in health care as well as other industries.[1–3] These systems vary accordingly to various design features (i.e. mandatory reporting, voluntary reporting, receiving reports from organizations, receiving reports from individuals, etc.). Each design feature may have certain advantages. For example, the advantages of receiving reports from organizations and from individuals are that they signify that the concerned institution has some commitment for making corrective system changes and also, the opportunity for input from frontline practitioners, respectively.

The scope of reporting systems may vary from one area to another. For example, the existing health care systems are generally narrow in focus and the non-healthcare ones are usually very comprehensive.

This chapter presents the various different aspects of health care human error reporting systems and related areas.

11.2   Effective Event-Reporting Systems and Approaches Practiced in Existing Reporting Systems

The effectiveness of event-reporting systems is a key element in order for them to be useful for the intended purposes such as making, say, health care systems less susceptible to human errors as well as reducing its overall cost. Although an effective reporting system has various key features, the two most important ones are as follows[4]:

- **Non-punitive.** It basically means that the people reporting error-related events are not subjected to any punishment. Past experiences indicate that this approach greatly facilitates reports of both actual events and "near-misses". For example, the National Aeronautics and Space Administration (NASA) Aviation Safety Reporting System (ASRS) grants automatic immunity for event reports received within ten days. Currently, the ASRS receives over 30000 event reports a year and it is regarded as a major factor in achieving remarkable safety of airplane travel in the United States.
- **Confidentiality.** It basically means that the identity of the reporting individuals or groups is kept secret. For example, in the case of ASRS after the verification of the event reports within a few days, the reports are "de-identified". More specifically, all traces of the sources of the information are removed to make it impossible to detect its origins in the future.

All in all, features such as these are important to be complemented by effective event-reporting systems in health care. Various experiences over the past 25 years in the aviation sector have shown that adverse event data, when carefully collected, analyzed, and interpreted, can help make the system not only less susceptible to human error but also less susceptible to design and operational failure as well.[5]

There are basically the following three approaches practiced in the existing event reporting systems[1]:

- **Approach I.** This involves mandatory reporting to an external entity. This approach is employed by the US States (e.g. California, Ohio, and Florida) that require reporting by health care facilities for accountability purposes.
- **Approach II.** This approach is voluntary and it reports confidentially to an external group for the purposes of improving quality. The current

medication reporting programs fall into this classification. Voluntary reporting systems are also used quite extensively in other industrial sectors, particularly in aviation.

- **Approach III.** This approach involves mandatory internal reporting with audit. A typical example of the approach, is the Occupational Safety and Health Administration (OSHA) approach that requires organizations to store data internally as indicated by the specified format. Then during any on-site inspections by OSHA the organizations will have these data readily available. Furthermore the internally kept data are not routinely submitted, but if the organization happened to be selected for an annual survey then these data have to be submitted as stated by the requirements.

11.3   Review of Current Human Error-Related Health Care Reporting Systems

Currently, there are many direct or indirect human-error related health care reporting systems in use. This section briefly reviews most of systems as follows[1]:

- **State Adverse Event Tracking Systems*.** These systems are used by various US state governments for the purpose of monitoring adverse events in health care organizations. Some of these systems have been in place for ten or more years. Two major impediments, cited for making greater use of the reported data in these systems, are the limitations in data and the lack of resources. All in all, it may be added that these systems appear to provide a public response for the investigation of certain events. However they are less likely to be successful in communicating concerns to the affected organizations or in synthesizing information to analyze where broad improvements might be needed.
- **Food and Drug Administration (FDA) Surveillance System.** As part of this system, reports are submitted to the FDA concerning adverse events associated with medical products after their formal approval.[6] In the case of medical devices, the manufacturers report information on areas such as malfunctions, serious injuries, and deaths. Furthermore user facilities such as nursing homes and hospitals are expected to report deaths to both the manufacturers and the FDA and also to report serious

---

*13 of these systems are discussed in detail later in the chapter.

injuries to the manufacturers. With respect to suspected adverse events concerning drugs, reporting is absolutely mandatory for the manufacturers, but in the case of physicians, consumers, etc. it is voluntary.

- **Joint Commission on Accreditation of Healthcare Organizations (JCAHO) Event Reporting System.** This is a sentinel event reporting system for hospitals and it was introduced by the JCAHO in 1996. A sentinel event may be defined as an unexpected occurrence or variation that involves death/serious psychological or physical injury/the risk thereof.[1] An organization experiencing a sentinel event is required by the JCAHO to perform the root cause analysis for the purpose of identifying event causal factors. Nonetheless, with regards to the reporting of the event to the JCAHO, a hospital may voluntarily report an incident and then submit the associated root cause analysis along with the proposed actions for improvement.[1]

- **Medication Errors Reporting System.** This is a voluntary medication error reporting system and it was originally developed by the Institute for Safe Medication Practice (ISMP) in 1975. Currently the system is managed by US Pharmacopoeia (USP) and it receives reports from frontline practitioners and shares its information with the FDA and the pharmaceutical companies.

- **MedMarx System.** This is an Internet-based, anonymous, voluntary system established for hospitals to report on medication errors. The system was established in 1998 by USP and its information is not shared with the FDA.

- **Mandatory Internal Reporting with Audit System.** This is basically an Occupational Safety and Health Administration (OSHA) requirement.[1,7] The requirement calls for the storage of internal records of injury and illness by companies employing eleven or more people. Although these companies are required to store internal records of injuries and illnesses, they are not required to submit the collected data routinely to the OSHA. When a company is included in the annual OSHA survey of companies, then it must have readily available injury and illness records for the on-site inspections.

- **Aviation Safety Reporting System (ASRS).** This is a non-medical, voluntary, and confidential incident reporting system. ASRS is used to highlight the hazards and latent system deficiencies so that they are eliminated or mitigated to improve system performance.[1] Although the ASRS was originally developed by the Federal Aviation Administration (FAA) in 1976, it is now funded only by the FAA, but is managed and operated by NASA. The system receives over 30000 incident-related reports per year and its annual operating budget is around \$2 million.[1]

All in all, it may be said that ASRS only maintains an effective database on reported incidents, performs analyses on the various types of incidents, highlights hazards and data patterns, and interview reporters when required. However, it has absolutely no regulatory powers over civil aviation.

Some of the key points associated with the existing event reporting systems are shown in Fig. 11.1.[1] Each of these point is briefly discussed. The effective reporting systems are useful also useful for their tools for error-related information gathering particularly from multiple reporters. In addition, they are ability to detect unusual features of the reporting systems.[8] The reporting systems are subjected to various challenges including getting sufficient participation in the programs and building an adequate response system.

The low occurrence of serious errors can lead to wide variations in frequency from one year to another as some organizations and individuals may routinely report more than the others due to various factors. There are minimal benefits of reporting systems without the adequate availability of resources for analysis and follow-up action. The heavy monitoring of medication errors by the various public and private reporting systems make it possible for a practitioner to voluntarily and confidentially report a medication error to the FDA or the other organizations. An effective feedback to the event reporters helps to influence the level of participation

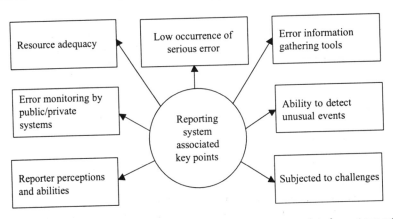

Fig. 11.1. Key points associated with the existing human error-related event reporting systems.

as it allows the reporters to perceive the benefits of reporting. More specifically to make the event reporters believe that the supplied information was actually used helps to assure them that the time spent in reporting events was worthwhile.

11.4   Lessons from Non-Medical Near Miss Reporting Systems

A near miss may simply be described as any event that could have had adverse consequences/events but it did not occur. Moreover, it is indistinguishable from fully fledged adverse events/consequences in all but the outcome.[9,10]

There are many near miss, "close call", or sentinel ("warning") event non-medical reporting systems being used in areas such as aviation, nuclear power generation, military, petrochemical processing, and steel production.[9] Over the years it has been observed that these systems which focus on near misses, provide good incentives for voluntary reporting. In addition they ensure reasonable confidentiality, and they emphasize the perspectives of systems on data gathering, analysis, and improvements to a certain degree.

There are many non-medical incidents reporting systems,[9] and Table 11.1 presents some of these systems.

Some of the common conflicts in near miss incident reporting systems are as follows[9]:

• Comparison of near miss data with accident data.

Table 11.1.   Selective non-medical incident reporting systems.

No.	System Name	Owned/Operated by
1	Aviation Safety Reporting System (ASRS)	National Aeronautics and Space Administration (NASA)
2	Confidential Human Factors Reporting System	British Airways
3	Human Factors Failure Analysis Classification System	US Navy and US Marines
4	Aviation Safety Airways Program	American Airlines
5	Air Safety Report	British Airways
6	Diagnostic Misadministration Reports-regulatory Information Distribution System	US Federal Government and Nuclear Regulatory Commission

Table 11.2. Barriers to event reporting by an individual.

No.	Barrier Type	Barrier(s)
1	Financial	Loss of job, reputation, etc.
2	Legal	Lack of trust, fear of reprisals, etc.
3	Regulatory	License suspension, increase in premiums, exposure to malpractice, etc.
4	Cultural	Fear of putting colleagues in trouble, code of silence, skepticism, etc.

Table 11.3. Incentives to event reporting by an individual.

No.	Incentive Type	Incentive(s)
1	Financial	Safety helps to save money.
2	Regulatory	Follow the rules.
3	Legal	Provide confidentiality and immunity.
4	Cultural	Integrity, professional values, educational, etc.

- Determining the right mix of barriers and incentives.
- Sacrificing accountability for information.
- Shift in focus from adverse events/errors to recovery processes.
- Trade off between national/large databases and regional systems.

Tables 11.2 and 11.3 present the barriers and incentives experienced in event reporting systems as compared to event reporting by an individual, respectively.

The organizational barriers and incentives to event reporting are presented in Tables 11.4 and 11.5, respectively.

11.5 State Adverse Medical Event Reporting Systems

A survey conducted by the Joint Commission on Accreditation of Healthcare Organizations (JCAHO) found that at least one-third of all US States have some form of adverse medical event reporting systems.[1,10] Several of these systems have been in place for over ten years and have undergone some forms of revisions since their inceptions. Generally, these reporting systems focus on patient injuries or facility issues and most of the time hospitals

Table 11.4.   Organizational barriers to event reporting.

No.	Barrier Type	Barrier(s)
1	Legal	Litigation fear, bad publicity, etc.
2	Financial	Potential loss of revenue, not cost effective, wastage of resources, etc.
3	Regulatory	"It does not apply to us", "we do our own internal analysis process", etc.
4	Cultural	Bureaucratic, dependent on organization, etc.

Table 11.5.   Organizational incentives to event reporting.

No.	Incentive Type	Incentive(s)
1	Financial	Improve reputation of safety and quality (good for business).
2	Regulatory	Fear of censure.
3	Legal	Provide confidentiality and immunity.
4	Cultural	Become a leader in safety and quality.

and/or nursing homes submit reports to these systems. Certain information reported to these systems is kept confidential with varying policies.

In particular, the survey revealed that the patient identifiers were never released, and the identity of the practitioner was rarely made available. For example, the state of Florida does not release any information that identifies any patients or hospitals; it releases only a statewide summary of the findings.

Table 11.6 presents some general information on adverse event reporting systems used in 13 US States.[1] Additional information on the reporting systems used by the 13 states is presented as follows[1]:

- **California**

  - **Reportable event.** This includes items such as major accidents, poisoning, epidemic outbreaks, deaths from unnatural causes, and other catastrophes and unusual occurrences that undermine the welfare of patients or others.

  - **Report submission.** Facilities such as general acute care hospitals, skilled nursing facilities, psychiatric hospitals, and psychology clinics are required to submit reports within 24 hours of the incident.

Table 11.6.   Some general information on reporting systems used in 13 states.

State Name	Initiation Year of the Reporting System	Reporting Requirement	Accumulated Number of Reports*
California	1972	Mandatory	4337 (1998)
Massachusetts	1986	Mandatory	10500 (1997)
Kansas	1986	Mandatory	488 (1997)
Rhode Island	1994	Mandatory	134 (1998)
Connecticut	1987	Mandatory for nursing homes, voluntary for hospitals	14783 (1996)
Colorado	1989	Mandatory	1233 (1998)
Florida	1985	Mandatory	Approximately 5000 reports per year
New York	1986	Mandatory	15000–20000 reports per year
New Jersey	1986	Mandatory	Unknown
Ohio	1997	Mandatory	Unknown
Pennsylvania	1990	Mandatory	Unknown
Mississippi	1993	Mandatory	Unknown
South Dakota	1994	Mandatory	Unknown

*The number in the parentheses indicates the year when the data were collected.

- **Access to information.** The reports containing non-confidential information are accessible to the general public. However, the reports containing confidential information can only be obtained through subpoena.

- Massachusetts

  - **Reportable event.** This includes medication errors, surgical errors, and injuries that is life-threatening, errors that results in death, or those requiring a patient to undergo significant treatments, etc.
  - **Report Submission.** All licensed health care facilities in the state are required to submit reports.
  - **Access to information.** After the action taken by the health department, reports are made available to public. However the reports concerning neglect, abuse, or misappropriation are classified as confidential; thus they are not released.

- **Kansas**
  - **Reportable event.** This includes an act by the health care provider that has a reasonable chance of causing injuries to patients, an act which is or may be below the standard of care, etc.
  - **Report submission.** All licensed health care facilities in the state are required to submit event reports.
  - **Access to information.** All submitted reports are considered confidential.

- **Rhode Island**
  - **Reportable event.** This includes any incident causing or incident involving items such as brain injuries, paralysis, impairment of hearing or sight, surgery on the wrong patient, and mental impairment.
  - **Report submission.** All hospitals in the state are required to submit the event reports.
  - **Access to information.** All submitted reports are considered confidential and are protected by the state law. Moreover the names of the individuals and the patients in the submitted reports are not disclosed.

- **Connecticut**
  - **Reportable event.** This includes all incidents/accidents that have caused deaths, serious injuries, or disruptions of facility services.
  - **Report submissions.** All nursing homes in the state are required to submit event reports. However, the submission of reports for hospitals is voluntary.
  - **Access to information.** Although the event reports disclose the name of the facility, information on individuals or patients is kept confidential.

- **Colorado**
  - **Reportable event.** This includes items such as deaths resulting from unexplained causes, transfusion errors, brain and spinal cord injuries, and the misuse of equipment.
  - **Report submission.** All licensed health care facilities functioning within the state are required to submit event reports.
  - **Access to information.** Although individual and patient information is kept confidential, the name of the facility is released.

- **Florida**
  - **Reportable event.** This includes urgent issues such as life-threatening situations, serious adverse events, and epidemic outbreak.

- **Report submission.** All hospitals and ambulatory surgical centers functioning in the state are required to submit event reports.
- **Access to information.** All information is kept confidential, but a summary of the aggregate data obtained from the reports is released on a yearly basis.

- **New York**

  - **Reportable event.** This is described as an unintended, undesirable, and adverse development in a patient's condition occurring in a hospital facility. Furthermore, the reportable event includes a list of 47 occurrences.
  - **Report submission.** All hospital facilities in the state are required to submit event reports.
  - **Access to information.** The aggregate data submitted by the hospitals, including the number of reports submitted can be released by the state. However the state law protects narrative reports on incidents and the investigations performed.

- **New Jersey**

  - **Reportable event.** This includes any incident that endangers the health and safety of an employee or patient as well as any fatalities or injuries relating to anesthetics.
  - **Report submission.** All licensed health care facilities functioning in the state are required to submit event reports.
  - **Access to information.** Although the patient and personnel information is kept confidential, other information is released when a facility receives a citation from the state.

- **Ohio**

  - **Reportable event.** This includes any fatalities/injuries caused by equipment failure or the treatment of the incorrect subject or the wrong modality.
  - **Report submission.** All functioning freestanding therapy, imaging, and chemotherapy centers in the state are required to submit event reports.
  - **Access to information.** The state law prohibits the collection of patient-related information and the state only releases aggregate data on the incident reported.

- **Pennsylvania**

  - **Reportable event.** This is described as any event that seriously compromises quality assurance or patient safety. It includes items such as deaths due to injuries, surgery on the wrong patient or modality, and deaths due to medication error.
  - **Report submission.** All hospitals, nursing homes, ambulatory surgical facilities, intermediate care facilities for persons with developmental disabilities, and nursing homes functioning in the state are required to submit event reports.
  - **Access to information.** All collected reports are considered confidential.

- **Mississippi**

  - **Reportable event.** This includes items such as wrongful death, interruptions of service at facility, unexplained injuries, abuse, and suicide or attempted suicide.
  - **Report submission.** All licensed health care facilities operating in the state are required to submit event reports.
  - **Access to information.** Although actual collected information is not accessible to the general public, statements of deficiencies and plans are made available upon request.

- **South Dakota**

  - **Reportable event.** This includes missing patients, incidents of neglect, abuse, or misappropriation, and unnatural deaths.
  - **Report submission.** All licensed health care facilities operating in the state are required to submit event reports.
  - **Access to information.** All reports are kept confidential, unless a below standard practice is highlighted at the health care facility. In such circumstances, a summary of the cited deficiency is considered releasable information.

All in all, the lack of resources and the limitations in data are cited as the two major factors for not having a greater use of the above reported data.

11.6   Human Error Data and Sources

Human error data play a critical role in making various types of human error occurrence decisions. Over the past 40 years, significant efforts have been made to collect and analyze various types of human error data.[11–12]. Although some of these data pertain to the medical field, a vast amount is concerned with non-medical areas. Nonetheless, some of these non-medical area data can also be used in making effective decisions in medicine.

This section presents various different aspects of human error data.

11.6.1   *Medical Human Error-Related Data*

Over the years various studies conducted in the medical field have generated various types of human error-related data. This section presents data directly or indirectly concerned with human error, generated by two distinct studies. Study I analyzed resident incident reports in a 703-bed hospital facility over a period of one year and has generated various types of quantitative data including the medication-related incident rates as presented in Table 11.7.[13]

Study II analyzed 30121 randomly selected records from 51 randomly selected acute care, non-psychiatric hospitals and has generated various types of data including rates of adverse events and negligence among clinical-specialty groups as presented in Table 11.8 and 11.9, respectively.[14]

11.6.2   *Non-Medical Human Error Data*

Over the past 40 years, a large amount of human error data in non-medical areas has been accumulated. Some of these data can also be used in medical areas. Table 11.10 presents the human error data for certain tasks/areas taken from published literature.[15–18]

Table 11.7.   Medication-related incident rates.

No.	Incident Description	Rate (Annual Incidence/100 beds)
1	Wrong medication administered.	3
2	Inappropriate dosing.	7
3	Medication administered without physician order.	1
4	Omission of dose.	5
5	Medication administered with known allergy.	0.14
6	Medication administered to wrong individual.	1

Table 11.8.   Adverse event rates for various clinical-specialty groups.

No.	Specialty Group	Adverse Event Rate (%)
1	General medicine	3.6
2	General surgery	7
3	Vascular surgery	16.1
4	Orthopedics	4.1
5	Obstetrics	1.5
6	Neurosurgery	9.9
7	Thoracic and cardiac surgery	10.8
8	Urology	4.9
9	Neonatology	0.6

Table 11.9.   Negligence rates for various clinical-specialty groups.

No.	Specialty Group	Negligence Rate (%)
1	General medicine	30.9
2	General surgery	28
3	Vascular surgery	18
4	Orthopedics	22.4
5	Obstetrics	38.3
6	Neurosurgery	35.6
7	Thoracic and cardiac surgery	23
8	Urology	19.4
9	Neonatology	25.8

11.6.3   *Human Error Data Sources*

Over the past four decades many human error-related data banks have been established and sources for obtaining such data have been identified. Some of these data banks and sources are as follows[1-3,19]:

- Aviation Safety Reporting System.[20]
- Data Store.[21]
- Air Force Inspection and Safety Center Life Science Accident and Incident Reporting System.[22]

Table 11.10. Human error occurrence probabilities for certain tasks/areas.

No.	Task/Error Description	Error Occurrence Probability
1	General error of omission.	0.01
2	Non-routine operation with other assigned responsibilities at the same time.	0.1
3	Normal oral communication.	0.03
4	General rate for errors involving very high stress.	0.3
5	Errors in simple arithmetic when self-checking as well.	0.03
6	Stressful complicated non-routine task.	0.3
7	Fast typing.	0.01
8	Keyphone dialing.	0.03
9	Use a checklist properly.	0.5
10	Read pressure gauge.	1.1×10^{-2}
11	Disconnect flexible hose.	1.9×10^{-3}
12	Error in a routine operation (where care is needed).	0.01
13	Error in simple routine operation.	0.001
14	Equipment turned in incorrect direction.	0.0002
15	Supervisor's failure to recognize the operator's error.	0.1
16	Incorrect switch (dissimilar in shape) selection.	0.001
17	Human-performance limit (single operator).	0.0001
18	Use written test/calibration procedures.	0.05
19	Install nuts, bolts, and plugs.	2×10^{-3}
20	Remove nuts, bolts, and plugs.	1.9×10^{-3}
21	Failure of operator to act in a correct manner after the first few hours under high stress conditions.	0.01
22	Use written maintenance procedures.	0.3
23	Install drain tube.	2×10^{-3}
24	Error of omission of an act entrenched in a procedure.	0.003
25	Failure of the operator to act in a correct manner in the first half-hour of a stressful emergency situation.	0.1
26	Remove drain tube.	1.9×10^{-3}
27	Position "zero-in" knob.	3.8×10^{-3}
28	General error rate for an act carried out wrongly.	0.003
29	Read flow/electrical meter.	1.4×10^{-2}
30	Connect flexible hose.	1.6×10^{-3}

- Nuclear Plant Reliability Data System.[23]
- Medication Errors Reporting (MER) Program.[1]
- Operational Performance Recording and Evaluation Data System.[24]
- Human Reliability: with Human Factors.[3]
- MedMarx (US Pharmacopoeia).[1]
- Safety Related Operator Action Program.[19]
- Bunker-ramo Tables.[25]
- Aerojet General Method.[17]

Problems

1. Write an essay on health care human error reporting systems.
2. Discuss the Aviation Safety Reporting System.
3. Describe the following two systems:

   - Food and Drug Administration Surveillance System.
   - Medication Errors Reporting (MER) System.

4. List the key points associated with the existing human error-related event reporting systems.
5. List at least five common conflicts in near miss incident reporting systems.
6. Define the term "near miss".
7. What is a state adverse medical event reporting system?
8. Discuss the adverse medical event reporting systems used by the following two states:

   - California
   - New York

9. Write down at least ten US States that have mandatory adverse medical event reporting systems.
10. List at least ten sources that can be used for obtaining human error-related data for application in medicine.

References

1. Kohn, L.T., Corrigan, J.M., and Donaldson, M.S., (eds), *To Err Is Human: Building a Safer Health System*, Institute of Medicine, National Academy Press, Washington, D.C., 1999.

2. Dhillon, B.S., *Human Reliability with Human Factors*, Pergamon Press, Inc., New York, 1986.
3. Dhillon, B.S., *Design Reliability: Fundamentals and Applications*, CRC Press, Inc., Boca Raton, Florida, 1999.
4. Spencer, F.C., "Human Error in Hospitals and Industrial Accidents: Current Concepts," *Journal of the American College of Surgeons*, Vol. 19, No. 14, 2000, pp. 410–418.
5. Billings, C.E., "Some Hopes and Concerns Regarding Medical Event-reporting Systems," *Arch. Path. Lab. Med.*, Vol. 122, 1998, pp. 214–215.
6. Food and Drug Administration (FDA), Washington, D.C.
7. *All about OSHA*, Report No. 2056, Occupational Safety and Health Administration (OSHA), Department of Labor, Washington, D.C., 1995.
8. Brewer, T. and Colditz, G.A., "Post-marketing Surveillance and Adverse Drug Reactions, Current Perspectives and Future Needs," *Journal of the American Medical Association (JAMA)*, Vol. 281, No. 9, 1999, pp. 824–829.
9. Barach, P. and Small, S.D., "Reporting and Preventing Medical Mishaps: Lessons from Non-medical Near Miss Reporting Systems," *British Medical Journal (BMJ)*, Vol. 320, 2000, pp. 759–763.
10. Barach, P., Small, S.D., and Kaplan, H., "Designing a Confidential Safety Reporting System: In Depth Review of Thirty Major Medical Incident Reporting Systems, and Near-miss Safety Reporting Systems in the Nuclear, Aviation, and Petrochemical Industries," *Anesthesiology*, Vol. 91, 1999, pp. A1209–A1220.
11. Williams, H.L., "Reliability Evaluation of the Human Component in Man-machine Systems," *Electrical Manufacturing*, April 1958, pp. 78–82.
12. Dhillon, B.S., "Human Error Data Banks," *Microelectronics and Reliability*, Vol. 30, 1990, pp. 963–971.
13. Gurwitz, J.H., Samchez-Cross, M.T., Eckler, M.S., *et al.*, "The Epidemiology of Adverse and Unexpected Events in the Long-term Care Setting," *Journal of the American Geriatric Society*, Vol. 42, 1994, pp. 33–38.
14. Brennan, T.A., Leape, L.L., Laird, N.M., *et al.*, "Incidence of Adverse Events and Negligence in Hospitalized Patients," *The New England Journal of Medicine*, Vol. 324, No. 6, 1991, pp. 370–376.
15. Kirwan, B., *A Guide to Practical Human Reliability Assessment*, Taylor and Francis Ltd., London, 1994.
16. Gertman, D.I. and Blackman, H.S., *Human Reliability and Safety Analysis Data Handbook*, John Wiley and Sons, New York, 1994.
17. Irwin, I.A., Levitz, J.J., and Freed, A.M., *Human Reliability in the Performance of Maintenance*, Report No. LRP317/TDR-63-218, Aerojet General Corporation, Sacramento, California, 1964.
18. Swain, A.D. and Guttmann, H.E., *Handbook of Human Reliability Analysis with Emphasis on Nuclear Power Plant Applications*, Report No. NUREG/CR-1278, US Nuclear Regulatory Commission, Washington, D.C., 1983.
19. Topmiller, D.A., Eckel, J.S., and Kozinsky, E.J., *Human Reliability Data Bank for Nuclear Power Plant Operations: A Review of Existing Human*

Reliability Data Banks, Report No. NUREG/CR2744/1, US Nuclear Regulatory Commission, Washington, D.C., 1982.

20. *Aviation Safety Reporting Program*, FAA Advisory Circular No. 00-46B, Federal Aviation Administration (FAA), Washington, D.C., 1979.

21. Munger, S.J., Smith, R.W., and Payne, D., *An Index of Electronic Equipment Operability: Data Store*, Report No. AIR-C43-1/62RP(1), American Institute for Research, Pittsburgh, Pennsylvania, 1962.

22. *Life Sciences Accident and Incident Classification Elements and Factors*, AFISC Operating Instruction No. AFISCM 127-6, US Air Force, Washington, D.C., 1971.

23. *Reporting Procedures Manual for the Nuclear Plant Reliability Data System* (NPRDS), South-West Research Institute, San Antonio, Texas, 1980.

24. Urmston, R., *Operational Performance Recording and Evaluation Data System (OPREDS)*, Descriptive Brochures, Code 3400, Navy Electronics Laboratory Center, San Diego, California, 1971.

25. Hornyak, S.J., *Effectiveness of Display Subsystems Measurement Prediction Techniques*, Report No. TR-67-292, Rome Air Development Center (RADC), Griffis Air Force Base, Rome, New York, 1967.

Appendix
Bibliography: Literature on Human Reliability and Error in Health Care

A.1 Introduction

Over the years, a large number of publications on human reliability/error in health care have appeared in the form of journal articles, conference proceedings articles, books, technical reports, and so on. This appendix presents a comprehensive list of these publications.

The period covered by list is from 1963 to 2000. The main objective of this listing is to provide readers with sources of additional information on human reliability and error in medical systems.

A.2 Publications

1. Abramson, N.S., Wald, K.S., Grenvik, A.A., and Robinson, D., "Adverse Occurrences in Intensive Care Units," *Journal of American Medical Association*, Vol. 244, No. 14, 1980, pp. 1582–1584.
2. Adams, J.G. and Bohan, S., "System Contributions to Error," *Academic Emergency Medicine*, Vol. 7, No. 11, 2000, pp. 1189–1193.
3. Alberti, K.G.M.M., "Medical Errors: A Common Problem," *British Medical Journal*, Vol. 322, Mar 2001, pp. 501–502.
4. Altshuler, C., Aster, R., Covino, K., Gordon, S., Gajewski, M., Smith, A., Horrigan, S., and Pfaff, K., "Automated Donor-recipient Identification Systems as a Means of Reducing Human Error in Blood Transfusion," *Transfusion*, Vol. 17, No. 6, 1977, pp. 586–597.
5. Andrews, L.B., Stocking, C., and Krizek, T., "An Alternative Strategy for Studying Adverse Events in Medical Care," *The Lancet*, Vol. 349, 1997, pp. 309–313.

6. Angelo, M. D., "Internet Solution Reduces Medical Errors," *Health Management Technology*, Feb 2000, pp. 20–21.

7. Apgar, B., "Patient Attitudes About Physician Mistakes," *American Family Physician*, Vol. 55, No. 6, 1997, pp. 2293–2295.

8. Arearese, J.S., "FDA's Role in Medical Device User Education," *The Medical Device Industry*, Estrin, N.F., (ed), Marcel Dekker Inc., New York, 1990, pp. 129–138.

9. Arnstein, F., "Catalogue of Human Error," *British Journal of Anaesthesia*, Vol. 79, 1997, pp. 645–656.

10. Baker, K.N. and Allan, E.L., "Research on Drug-use-system Errors," *American Journal of Health System Pharmacy*, Vol. 52, 1995, pp. 400–403.

11. Barach, P. and Small, S. D., "Reporting and Preventing Medical Mishaps: Lessons from Non-medical Near Miss Reporting Systems," *British Medical Journal*, Vol. 320, 2000, pp. 759–763.

12. Bates, D.W., Cullen, D.J., Small, S.D., Cooper, J.B., Nemeskal, A.R., and Leape, L.L., "The Incident Reporting System Does Not Detect Adverse Drug Events: A Problem for Quality Improvement," *Joint Commission Journal on Quality Improvement*, Vol. 21, No. 10, 1995, pp. 541–548.

13. Bates, D. W., Spell, N., and Cullen, D. J., "The Costs of Adverse Drug Events in Hospitalized Patients." *Journal of American Medical Association*, Vol. 277, No. 4, 1997, pp. 307–311.

14. Bates, D. W., "Using Information Technology to Reduce Rates of Medication Errors in Hospitals," *British Medical Journal*, Vol. 320, 2000, pp. 788–791.

15. Bates, D.W., O'Neil, A.C., and Boyle, D., "Potential Identifiability and Preventability of Adverse Events Using Information Systems," *Journal of the American Informatics Association*, Vol. 5, 1994, pp. 404–411.

16. Battles, J.B., Kaplan, H.S., Van der Schaaf, T.W., and Shea, C.E., "The Attributes of Medical Event-reporting Systems," *Archives of Pathology and Laboratory Medicine*, Vol. 122, 1998, pp. 231–238.

17. Battles, J., Mercer, Q., Whiteside, M., and Bradley, J., "A Medical Event Reporting System for Human Errors in Transfusion Medicine," Ozok A.F. & Salvendy G., (eds), *Advances in Applied Ergonomics*, USA Publishing, West Lafayette, 1996, pp. 809–814.

18. Battles, J, Mercer, Q., Whiteside, M., and Bradley, J., "Human Errors in Transfusion Medicine: Multi-disciplinary Design of an Ideal Event Reporting System," Ozok A.F. and Salvendy G., (eds), *Advances in Applied Ergonomics*, USA Publishing, West Lafayette, 1996, pp. 782–787.

19. Battles, J, Mercer, Q., Whiteside, M., and Bradley, J., "Using the Delphi Method to Design an Ideal Error Reporting System for the Blood Transfusion Process," *Proceedings of the 59th Annual Meeting of the American Society for Information Science*, Baltimore, Maryland, 1996, pp. 116–125.

20. Baylis, F., "Errors in medicine: Nurturing Truthfulness," *Journal of Clinical Ethics*, Vol. 8, 1997, pp. 336–340.

21. Beckmann, U., Baldwin, I., Hart, G.K., and Runciman, W.B., "The Australian Incident Monitoring Study in Intensive Care: AIMS-ICU, An

Analysis of the First Year of Reporting," *Anaesthetic Intensive Care*, Vol. 24, 1996, pp. 320–329.

22. Beckmann, U., West, L.F., Groombridge, G.J., and Webb, R.K., "The Australian Incident Monitoring Study in Intensive Care: AIMS-ICU. The Development and Evaluation of an Incident Reporting System in Intensive Care," *Anaesthesia and Intensive Care*, Vol. 24, No. 3, 1996, pp. 314–319.

23. Beith, B.H., "Human Factors and the Future of Telemedicine," *Medical Device & Diagnostic Industry Magazine*, Vol. 21, No. 6, 1999, pp. 36–40.

24. Belkin, L., "Human and Mechanical Failures Plague Medical Care," *The New York Times*, March 31, 1992, pp. B1 and B6.

25. Bell, B.M., "Error in Medicine," *Journal of American Medical Association*, Vol. 274, No. 6, 1995, pp. 457–461.

26. Berglund, S., "Systems Failures, Human Error and Health Care," *Medical Liability Monitor*, 1998, pp. 1–4.

27. Billings, C.E. and Woods, D.D., "Human Error in Perspective: The Patient Safety Movement," *Postgraduate Medicine*, Vol. 109, No. 1, 2001. pp. 23–25.

28. Billings, C.E., "Some Hopes and Concerns Regarding Medical Event-reporting Systems: Lessons from the NASA Aviation Safety Reporting System," *Archives of Pathology and Laboratory Medicine*, Vol. 122, No. 3, 1998, pp. 214–215.

29. Bindler, R. and Boyne, T., "Medication Calculation Ability of Registered Nurses, *Image*, Vol. 23, 1991, pp. 221–224.

30. Blumenthal, D., "Making Medical Errors into Medical Treasures," *Journal of American Medical Association*, Vol. 272, No. 23, 1994, pp. 1867–1869.

31. Beiser, E.N., "Reporting Physicians' Mistakes," *Rhode Island Medical Journal*, Vol. 73, No. 8, 1990, pp. 333–336.

32. Bogner, M.S., "Medical Device and Human Error," *Human Performance in Automated Systems: Current Research and Trends*, Mouloua, M., and Parasuraman, P., (eds), Hillsdale, Lawrence Erlbaum Associates Publishers, Hillsdale, New Jersey, 1994, pp. 64–67.

33. Bogner, M.S., "Technology and Human Error in Medicine," *Conference Proceedings of the SPIE*, Vol. 32, 1995, pp. 374–384.

34. Bogner, M.S., "Human Error in Medicine," *Human Error in Medicine*, Bogner, M.S., (ed), Lawrence Erlbaum Associates Publishers, Hillsdale, New Jersey, 1994, pp. 373–385.

35. Bogner, M.S., "Human Factors, Human Error and Patient Safety Panel," *Proceedings of the Annual Human Factors Society Conference*, Vol. 2, 1998, pp. 1053–1057.

36. Bogner, M.S., "Designing Medical Devices to Reduce the Likelihood of Error," *Biomedical Instrumentation and Technology*, Vol. 33, No. 2, 1999, pp. 108–113.

37. Bogner, M.S., "Medical Device: A Frontier for Human Factors," *CSERIAC Gateway*, Vol. 4, No. 1, 1993, pp. 12–14.

38. Botney, R. and Gaba, D.M., "Human Factors Issues in Monitoring, Blitt, C.D and Hines, R.L., (ed), *Monitoring in Anesthesia and Critical Care Medicine*, Churchill Livingstone Publications, New York, 1997, pp. 23–54.

39. Bracco, D., Favre, J. B., and Bissonnette, B., "Human Errors in a Multidisciplinary Intensive Care Unit: A 1-Year Prospective Study," *Intensive Care Med*, Vol. 27, 2001, pp. 137–145.

40. Bradley, J.B., "Controlling Risk in a Complex Environment: The Design of Computer-based Systems to Minimize Human Error in Medicine," *Proceedings of the ASIS Annual Conference*, October, 1996, pp. 210–213.

41. Brady, W.J. and Perron, A., "Errors in Emergency Physician Interpretation of ST-Segment Elevation in Emergency Department Chest Pain Patients," *Academic Emergency Medicine*, Vol. 7, No. 11, 2000, pp. 1256–1260.

42. Brasel, K.J., Layde, P.M., and Hargarten, S., "Evaluation of Error in Medicine: Application of a Public Health Model," *Academic Emergency Medicine*, Vol. 7, No. 11, 2000, pp. 1298–1302.

43. Bratman, R.L., "A National Database of Medical Error," *Journal of Royal Society of Medicine*, Vol. 93, 2000, p. 106.

44. Brazeau, C., "Disclosing the Truth About a Medical Error," *American Family Physician*, Vol. 60, 1999, pp. 1013–1014.

45. Brennan, S.L., "Disclosure of Error and the Threat of Malpractice," *Ethical Choices: Case Studies for Medical Practice*, American College of Physicians, Philadelphia, March 1996.

46. Brennan, T.A., Leape, L.L., and Laird, N.M., "Incidence of Adverse Events and Negligence in Hospitalized Patients: Results of the Harvard Medical Practice Study II," *The New England Journal of Medicine*, Vol. 324, 1991, pp. 377–384.

47. Brennan, T.A., Localio, R., Leape, L.L., and Laird, N.M., "Identification of Adverse Events Occurring During Hospitalization," *Annals of Internal Medicine*, Vol. 112, No. 3, 1990, pp. 221–226.

48. Brennan, T.A., "The Institute of Medical Report on Medical Errors—Could It Do Harm," *The New England Journal of Medicine*, Vol. 342, No. 15, 2000, pp. 1123–1125.

49. Brennan, T.A., Jocalio, R.J., and Laird, N.L., "Reliability and Validity of Judgements Concerning Adverse Events Suffered by Hospitalized Patients," *Medical Care*, Vol. 27, No. 12, 1989, pp. 1148–1158.

50. Brennan, T.A., Leape, L.L., and Laird, N.M., "Incidence of Adverse Events and Negligence in Hospitalized Patients: Results of the Harvard Medical Practice Study-I," *The New England Journal of Medicine*, Vol. 324, 1991, pp. 370–376.

51. Brennan, T.A., Bates, D.W., Pappius, E., Kuperman, G.J., Sittig, D., Burstin, H., Fairchild, D., and Teich, J.M., "Using Information Systems to Measure and Improve Quality," *International Journal of Medical Informatics*, Vol. 53, No. 2–3, 1999, pp. 115–124.

52. Brienza, J., "Medical Mistakes Study Highlights Need for System Wide Improvements," *Trail*, February 2000, pp. 15–17.

53. Brooke, P.S., "Shaping the Medical Error Movement," *Nursing Management*, Vol. 31, No. 8, 2000, pp. 18–19.

54. Brown, S.L., Bogner, M.S., Parmentier, C.M., and Taylor, J.B., "Human Error and Patient-controlled Analgesia Pumps," *Journal of Intravenous Nursing*, Vol. 20, No. 6, 1997, pp. 311–316.

55. Brown, R.W., "Errors in Medicine," *Journal of Quality Clinical Practice*, Vol. 17, 1997, pp. 21–25.

56. Bruley, M.E., "Ergonomics and Error: Who is Responsible," *Proceeding of the First Symposium on Human Factors in Medical Devices*, 1989, pp. 6–10.

57. Bruno, K.J., Welz, L.L., and Sherif, J., "Developing an Error Prevention Methodology Based on Cognitive Error Models," *Proceedings of ACM CHI'92 Conference on Human Factors in Computing Systems — Posters and Short Talks*, Vol. 53, 1992.

58. Burlington, D.B., "Human Factors and the FDA's Goal: Improved Medical Device Design," *Biomedical Instrumentation & Technology*, Vol. 30, No. 2, 1996, pp. 107–109.

59. Busse, D.K. and Wright, D.J., "Classification and Analysis of Incidents in Complex, Medical Environment," *Topics in Health Information Management*, Vol. 20, No. 4, 2000, pp. 56–58.

60. Busse, D.K. and Johnson, C.W., "Human Error in an Intensive Care Unit B: A Cognitive Analysis of Critical Incidents," *Proceedings of the 17th International Conference of the Systems Safety Society*, Orlando, Florida, USA, August 1999, pp. 70–75.

61. Busse, D.K. and Johnson, C.W., "Modeling Human Error Within a Cognitive Theoretical Framework," *Proceedings of the 2nd European Conference of Cognitive Modelling (ECCM-98)*, Ritter, F.E., and Young, R.M., (eds), Nottingham University Press, Nottingham, 1998, pp. 90–97.

62. Busse, D.K. and Johnson, C.W., "Using a Cognitive Theoretical Framework to Support Accident Analysis," *Proceedings of the 2nd Workshop on Human Error, Safety, and Systems Development*, Seattle, April 1998, pp. 10–15.

63. Caldwell, R., Alerting Staff to Medication Errors, *Health Management Technology*, August 2000, p. 52.

64. Caplan, R.A., Vistica, M.F., Posner, K.L., and Cheney, F.W., "Adverse Anaesthetic Outcomes Arising from Gas Delivery Equipment: A Closed Claims Analysis," *Anaesthesiology*, Vol. 87, No. 4, 1997, pp. 741–748.

65. Carnall, D., "Error in Medicine," *British Medical Journal*, Vol. 320, 2000, p. 811.

66. Casey, S., *Set Phasers on Stun: and Other True Tales of Technology and Human Error*, Argean, Inc., Santa Barbara, California, 1993.

67. Casarett, D. and Helms, C., "Systems Errors versus Physicians' Errors: Finding the Balance in Medical Education," *Academic Medicine*, Vol. 74, 1999, pp. 19–22.

68. Cattaneo, C.R. and Vecchio, A.D., "Human Errors in the Calculation of Monitor Units in Clinical Radiotherapy Practice," *Radiotherapy and Oncology*, Vol. 28, No. 1, 1993, pp. 86–88.

69. Charatan, F., "Clinton Acts to Reduce Medical Mistakes," *British Medical Journal*, Vol. 320, 2000, p. 597.

70. Chassin, M.R. and Galvin, R.W., "The Urgent Need to Improve Health Care Quality," *Journal of American Medical Association*, Vol. 280, 1998, pp. 1000–1005.

71. Chassin, M.R., "Is Health Care Ready for Six Sigma Quality," *The Milbank Quarterly-J, of Public Health and Health Care Policy*, Vol. 76, No. 4, 1998, pp. 59–61.

72. Chopra, V., Bovill, J.G., and Koornneef, J.F., "Reported Significant Observations During Anaesthesia: A Prospective Analysis Over a 18-month Period," *British Journal of Anaesthesia*, Vol. 68, 1992, pp. 13–17.

73. Christakis, N.A. and Lamont, E.B., "Extent and Determinants of Error in Doctors' Prognoses in Terminally Ill Patients: Prospective Cohort Study," *British Medical Journal*, Vol. 320, 2000, pp. 469–473.

74. Christensen, J.F., Levinson, W., and Dunn, P.M., "The Heart of Darkness: The Impact of Perceived Mistakes on Physicians," *Journal of General Internal Medicine*, Vol. 7, 1992, pp. 424–431.

75. Clarke, J.C., Spejewski, B., Gertner, A.S., Webber, B.L., Catherine Z., Hayward, C.Z., and Santora, T.A., "An Objective Analysis of Process Errors in Trauma Resuscitations," *Academic Emergency Medicine*, Vol. 7, No. 11, 2000, pp. 1303–1310.

76. Classen, D., "Patient Safety, the Name is Quality," *Trustee*, Vol. 53, No. 9, 2000, pp. 12–15.

77. Clifton, B.S. and Hotten, W.I.T., "Deaths Associated with Anaesthesia," *British Journal of Anaesthesia*, Vol. 35, 1963, pp. 250–259.

78. Cohen, M.R., Senders, J., and Davis, N.M., "Failure Mode and Effects Analysis: a Novel Approach to Avoiding Dangerous Medication Errors and Accidents," *Hospital Pharmacy*, Vol. 29, No. 4, 1994, pp. 319–330.

79. Cole, T., "Medical Errors vs Medical Injuries: Physicians Seek to Prevent Both," *Journal of American Medical Association*, Vol. 284, No. 17, November 1, 2000, pp. 2175–2176.

80. Coleman, I.C. and Pharm, D., "Medication Errors: Picking up the Pieces," *Drug Topics*, March 15, 1999, pp. 83–92.

81. Conlan, M.F., "IOM's Med-error Report Spurs Changes Among Pharmacies, *Drug Topics*, Vol. 144, No. 23, 2000, pp. 70–71.

82. Conlan, M.F., "Tasks Force Starts Shaping Research to Cut Med Errors," *Drugs Topics*, October 2000, p. 69.

83. Cook, R.I. and Woods, D.D., "A Tale of Two Stories: Contrasting Views of Patient Safety," *Report from a Workshop on Assembling the Scientific Basis for Progress on Patient Safety*, National Health Care Safety Council of the National Patient Safety Foundation at the AMA, Chicago, Illinois, 2000.

84. Cook, R.I. and Woods, D.D., "Operating at the Sharp End: The Complexity of Human Error," *Human Error in Medicine*, Bogner, M.S., (ed), Lawrence Erlbaum Associates Publishers, Hillsdale, New Jersey, 1994, pp. 255–310.

85. Cooper, J.B., "Toward Prevention of Anaesthetic Mishaps," *International Anesthesiology Clinics*, Vol. 22, 1985, pp. 167–183.

86. Cooper, D.M., "Series of Errors Led to 300 Unnecessary Mastectomies," *British Medical Journal*, Vol. 320, 2000, p. 597.

87. Cooper, J.B. and Gaba, D.M., "A Strategy for Preventing Anaesthesia Accidents," *International Anesthesiology Clinics*, Vol. 27, No. 3, 1989, pp. 148–152.

88. Cooper, J.B., Newbower, R.S., and Kitz, R.J., "An Analysis of Major Errors and Equipment Failures in Anaesthesia Management: Consideration for Prevention and Detection," *Anaesthesiology*, Vol. 60, No. 1, 1984, pp. 34–42.

89. Cooper, J.B., Newbower, R.S., Long, C.D., and McPeek, B., "Preventable Anaesthesia Mishaps" *Anaesthesiology*, Vol. 49, 1978, pp. 399–406.

90. Cott V.H., "Human Error: Their Causes and Reduction," *Human Error in Medicine*, Bogner, M.S., (ed), Lawrence Erlbaum Associates Publishers, Hillsdale, New Jersey, 1994, pp. 53–65.

91. Craig, J. and Wilson, M.E., "A Survey of Anaesthetic Misadventures," *Anaesthesia*, Vol. 36, 1981, pp. 933–936.

92. Crane, M., "How Good Doctors Can Avoid Bad Errors," *Medical Economics*, April 28, 1997, pp. 36–43.

93. Cullen, D.J., "Risk Modification in the Post Anaesthesia Care Unit," *International Anaesthesia Clinics*, Vol. 27, No. 3, 1989, pp. 184–187.

94. Curtin, L. and Simpson, R. L., "Quality of Care and the Low Hanging Fruit," *Health Management Technology*, Vol. 21, No. 9, 2000, pp. 48–49.

95. David, B.D., Favre, J.B., Bissonnette, B., Wasserfallen, J.B., Revelly, J.P., and Ravussin, P., "Human Errors in a Multidisciplinary Intensive Care Unit: A 1-Year Prospective Study," *Intensive Care Medicine*, Vol. 32, 1998, pp. 569–573.

96. David, P.P., Glyyn, C.N., and Laura, M., "Increase in US Medication-error Deaths Between 1983–1993, *Lancet*, Vol. 351, 1998, pp. 643–644.

97. Davis, J.M. and Strunin, L., "Anaesthesia in 1984: How Safe is it," *Canadian Medical Association Journal*, Vol. 131, 1984, pp. 437–441.

98. Davis, N. and Cohen, M., "Medication Errors: Causes and Prevention," N.M. Davis Association, Huntingdon Valley, Pennsylvania, 1983.

99. Davis, J.W., Hoyt, D.B., and McArdle, M.S., "The Significance of Critical Care Errors in Causing Preventable Death in Trauma Patients in a Trauma Station," *Journal of Trauma*, Vol. 31, 1991, pp. 813–819.

100. De Leval, M.R., "Human Factors and Surgical Outcomes: a Cartesian Dream," *The Lancet*, Vol. 349, No. 9053, 1997, pp. 723–726.

101. De Leval, M.R. and Reason, J.T., "The Human Factor in Cardiac Surgery: Errors and Near Misses in a High Technology Medical Domain," *Annals of Thoracic Surgery*, Vol. 72, No. 1, 2001, pp. 300–305.

102. DeAnda, A. and Gaba, D.M., "Unplanned Incidents During Comprehensive Anaesthesia Simulation," *Anaesthesia Analgesia*, Vol. 71, 1990, pp. 77–82.

103. "Deaths During General Anesthesia: Technology-related, Due to Human Error, or Unavoidable? An ECRI Technology Assessment," *Journal of Health Care Technology*, Vol. 1, No. 3, 1985, pp. 155–175.

104. Davidson, J.S., "Errors in Emergency Medicine: Not Quite Random Ruminations of a Curmudgeon," *Academic Emergency Medicine*, Vol. 7, No. 11, 2000, pp. 1334–1337.

105. Dhillon, B.S., "Human Error in Medical Systems," *Proceedings of the 6th ISSAT International Conference on Reliability and Quality in Design*, 2000, pp. 138–143.

106. Dhillon, B.S., "Human Error in Health Care Systems," *Medical Device Reliability and Associated Area*, CRC Press, Boca Raton, Florida, 2000, pp. 51–68.

107. Domizio, G.D., Davis, N.M., and Cohen, M.R., "The Growing Risk of Look-alike Trademarks," *Medical Marketing and Media*, May 1992, pp. 24–30.

108. Donchin, Y., Gopher, D., Olin, M., and Badihi, Y., "A Look into the Nature and Causes of Human Error in the Intensive Care Unit," *Critical Care Medicine*, Vol. 23, No. 2, 1995, pp. 294–300.

109. Dorevitch, S. and Frost, L., "The Occupational Hazards of Emergency Physicians," *American Journal Emergency Medicine*, Vol. 18, No. 3, 2000, pp. 300–311.

110. Doyal, L., "The Mortality of Medical Mistakes, Doctors-obligations and Patients-expectation," *The Practitioner*, Vol. 231, 1987, pp. 615–620.

111. Dripps, R.D., Lamont, A., and Eckenhoff, J.E., "The Role of Anesthesia in Surgical Mortality," *Journal of American Medical Association*, Vol. 178, 1991, pp. 261–266.

112. Dunn, J.D., "Error in Medicine," *Annuls of Internal Medicine*, Vol. 134, No. 4, 2001, pp. 342–344.

113. Dutton, G., "Do American Hospitals Get Away with Murders," *Business and Health*, Vol. 18, No. 4, 2000, pp. 38–47.

114. Dyer, C., "Study Identifies why Child Heart Operations Go Wrong," *British Medical Journal*, Vol. 319, 1999, p. 803.

115. Editorial, "Promoting Patient Safety by Preventing Medical Error," *Journal of American Medical Association*, Vol. 280, No. 16, 1998, pp. 1444–1148.

116. Egger, E., "Medical Errors: It Pays for Hospitals to Support Programs that Help Control Physician Stress," *Health Care Strategic Management*, March 2000, pp. 18–19.

117. Eisele, G.R. and Watkins, J.P., *"Survey of Workplace Violence in Department of Energy Facilities,"* A Report Prepared for US Department of Energy, Office of Occupational Medicine and Medical Surveillance, Washington, D.C., December 1995.

118. Eisenberg, J.M., "The Best Offence is a Good Defence Against Medical Errors: Putting the Full-court Press on Medical Errors," *Agency for Health-care Research and Quality*, Duke University Clinical Research Institute, Rockville, Maryland, January 20, 2000.

119. Eisenberg, J.M., "Medical Error Accountability," *Family Practice News*, Vol. 30, No. 9, 2000, p. 12.

120. Eisenberg, J.M., "Medical Errors and Patient Safety: a Growing Research Priority," *Health Services Research*, Chicago, Illinois, Vol. 35, No. 3, 2000, pp. 11–16.

121. Eisenberg, J.M., "Statement on Medical Errors," *Report Before the Senate Appropriations Subcommittee on Labor, Health and Human Services, and Education*, Washington, D.C., USA, December 13, 1999.

122. Epstein, R.M., "Morbidity and Mortality from Anaesthesia," *Anaesthesiology*, Vol. 49, 1978, pp. 388–389.

123. Espinosa, J.A. and Nolan, T.W., "Reducing Errors Made by Emergency Physician in Interpreting Radiographs: Longitudinal Study," *British Medical Journal*, Vol. 320, 2000, pp. 737–740.

124. Famularo, G., Salvani, P., and Terranova, A., "Clinical Errors in Emergency Medicine: Experience at the Emergency Department of an Italian Teaching Hospital," *Academic Emergency Medicine*, Vol. 7, No. 11, 2000, pp. 1278–1281.

125. Feinstein, A.R., "Errors in Getting and Interpreting Evidence," *Perspectives in Biology and Medicine*, Vol. 41, No. 1, 1999, pp. 45–58.

126. Feldman, S.E. and Roblin, D.W., "Medical Accidents in Hospitals Care: Applications of Failure Analysis to Hospitals Quality Appraisal," *Journal of Quality Improvement*, Vol. 23, No. 11, 1997, pp. 567–580.

127. Ferman, J., "Medical Errors Spur New Patient — Safety Measures," *Healthcare Executive*, March 2000, pp. 55–56.

128. Ferner, R.E., "Reporting of Critical Incidents Shows How Errors Occur," *British Medical Journal*, Vol. 311, 1995, p. 1368.

129. Ferner, R.E., "Medication Errors that have Led to Manslaughter Charges," *British Medical Journal*, Vol. 321, 2000, pp. 1212–1216.

130. Fisher, M.J., "Eliminating Medical Errors is Sound Risk Management," *National Underwriter*, October 5, 1998, p. 51.

131. Flickinger, J.C. and Lunsford, L.D., "Potential Human Error in Setting Stereo Tactic Coordinates for Radiotherapy: Implication for Quality Assurance," *International Journal of Radiation Oncology, Biology, Physics*, Vol. 27, No. 2, 1993, pp. 397–401.

132. Fox, G.N., "Minimizing Prescribing Errors in Infants and Children," *American Family Physician*, Vol. 53, No. 4, 1996, pp. 1319–1325.

133. Furness, P.N. and Lauder, I., "A Questionnaire-based Survey of Errors in Diagnostic Histopathology Throughout the United Kingdom," *Journal of Clinical Pathology*, Vol. 50, 1997, pp. 457–460.

134. Gaba, D.M., "Anaesthesiology as a Model for Patient Safety in Healthcare," *British Medical Journal*, Vol. 320, 2000, pp. 785–788.

135. Gaba, D.M. and Maxwell, M., "Anaesthetic Mishaps: Breaking the Chain of Accidents Evolution," *Anaesthesiology*, Vol. 66, 1987, pp. 670–675.

136. Gaba, D.M., "Human Error in Anaesthetic Mishaps," *International Anaesthesiology Clinics*, Vol. 27, No. 3, 1989, pp. 137–147.

137. Gaba, D.M., "Human Error in Dynamic Medical Domains," *Human Error in Medicine*, Bogner, M.S., (ed), Lawrence Erlbaum Associates Publishers, Hillsdale, NJ, 1994, pp. 197–224.

138. Gaba, D.M. and Howard S.K., "Conference on Human Error in Anaesthesia (meeting report)," *Anaesthesiology*, Vol. 75, 1991, pp. 553–554.

139. Gaba, D.M., "Human Performance Issues in Anaesthesia Patient Safety," *Problems in Anaesthesia*, Vol. 5, 1991, pp. 329–330.

140. Gawande, A.A., Thomas, E.J., and Zinner, M.J., "The Incidence and Nature of Surgical Adverse Events in Colorado and Utah in 1992," *Surgery*, Vol. 126, No. 1, 1999, pp. 66–75.

141. Gebhart, F., "Hospitals-VHA and VA-alike Launch Programs to Cut Errors," *Drug Topics*, November 20, 2000, p. 53.
142. George, D., "A Medical Error," *British Medical Journal*, Vol. 320, 2000, p. 1283.
143. Gerlin, A., "Medical Mistakes," *The Inquirer*, September 12, 1999, pp. 64–65.
144. Glick, T.H., Workman, T.P., and Gaufrerg, S. V., "Human Error in Medicine," *Academic Emergency Medicine*, Vol. 7, No. 11, 2000, pp. 1272–1277.
145. Gopher, D., Olin, M., and Badihi, Y., "The Nature and Causes of Human Errors in a Medical Intensive Care Unit," *Proceedings of the Human Factors Society 33rd Annual Meeting*, 1989, pp. 956–960.
146. Gorman, C., "The Disturbing Case of the Cure that Killed the Patient," *Time*, 3 April, 1995, pp. 60–61.
147. Gosbee, J., "Importance of Human Factors Engineering in Error and Medicine Education," *Academic Medicine*, Vol. 74, No. 7, 1999, pp. 748–749.
148. Grasha, A.F., "Into the Abyss: Seven Principles for Identifying the Causes of and Preventing Human Error in Complex Systems," *American Journal of Health System Pharmacy*, Vol. 57, No. 6, 2000, pp. 554–564.
149. Gravenstein, J.S., "How Does Human Error Affect Safety in Anesthesia?," *Surgical Oncology Clinics of North America*, Vol. 9, No. 1, 2000, pp. 81–95.
150. Green, R., "The Psychology of Human Error," *European Journal of Anaesthesiology*, Vol. 16, No. 3, 1999, pp. 148–155.
151. Greene, J., "True Fix-medical Errors," *Hospitals & Health Network*, February 2000, pp. 55–59.
152. Gunn, I.P., "Patient Safety and Human Error: The Big Picture," *CRNA*, Vol. 11, No. 1, 2000, pp. 41–48.
153. Gurwitz, J.H., Sanchez-Cross, M.T., Eckler, M.A., and Matulis, J., "The Epidemiology of Adverse and Unexpected Events in the Long-term Care Setting," *Journal of the American Geriatric Society*, Vol. 42, 1994, pp. 33–38.
154. Hallam, K., "An Erosion of Trust: Survey Finds Consumers Fear Medical Errors and Want Better Protection From Such Mistakes," *Modern Healthcare*, Vol. 30, No. 52, 2000, pp. 30–31.
155. Handler, J.A., Gillam, M., and Sanders, A.B., "Defining, Identifying, and Measuring Medical Error in Emergency Medicine," *Academic Emergency Medicine*, Vol. 7, No. 11, 2000, pp. 1183–1188.
156. Harrison, B.T., Gibberd, R.W., and Hamilton, J.D., "An Analysis of the Causes of Adverse Events from the Quality in Australian Health Care Study," *Medical Journal of Australia*, Vol. 170, No. 9, 1999, pp. 411–415.
157. Hart G.K., Baidwin, I., Ford, J., and Gutteridge, G.A., "Adverse Incidents in Intensive Care Survey," *Anaesthesia and Intensive Care*, Vol. 21, No. 5, 1993, pp. 65–68.
158. Hatlie, M.J., Scapegoating Won't Reduce Medical Errors, *Medical Economics*, Vol. 77, No. 10, 2000, pp. 92–100.

159. Hearnshaw, H., "Human Error in Medicine," *Ergonomics*, Vol. 39, No. 6, 1996, pp. 899–900.

160. Hector, J. and Tom, P., "Missed Diagnosis of Acute Cardiac Ischemia in the Emergency Department," *New England Journal of Medicine*, Vol. 342, 2000, pp. 1163–1170.

161. Helmreich, R.L. and Schaefer, H. G., "Team Performance in the Operating Room," *Human Error in Medicine*, Bogner, M.S., (ed), Lawrence Erlbaum Associates Publishers, Hillsdale, New Jersey, 1994, pp. 225–254.

162. Helmreich, R.L., "On Error Management: Lessons From Aviation," *British Medical Journal*, Vol. 320, 2000, pp. 781–785.

163. Dhillon, B.S., "Human Error in Health Care System," in *Medical Device Reliability and Associated Areas*, CRC Press, Boca Raton, Florida, 2000, pp. 51–68.

164. Hobgood, C.D., John, O., and Swart, L., "Emergency Medicine Resident Errors: Identification and Educational Utilization," *Academic Emergency Medicine*, Vol. 7, No. 11, 2000, pp. 1317–1320.

165. Hollnagel, E., *Cognitive Reliability and Error Analysis*, Elsevier publishers, Amsterdam, 1998.

166. Hollnagel, E., Kaarstad, M., and Lee, H.C., "Error Mode Prediction," *Ergonomics*, Vol. 42, No. 11, 1999, pp. 1457–1471.

167. Horan, S., "Is Human Error the Cause of Accident and Disaster?," *Occupational Health*, Vol. 45, No. 5, 1993, pp. 169–172.

168. "How Safe is our Healthcare System? What States Can do to Improve Patient Safety and Reduce Medical Errors," *Proceedings of a Workshop Sponsored by the Agency for Healthcare Research and Quality (AHRQ)*, Boston, Massachusetts, 2000, pp. 20–25.

169. "How States can Improve Patient Safety and Reduce Medical Errors," Transcript of part two of the series of National Audio Teleconferences sponsored by the User Liaison Program, *Agency for Healthcare Research and Quality*, Rockville, Maryland, conducted on May 24, 2000.

170. Hughes, C.M., Honig, P., Phillips, J., Woodcook, J., Richard E. Anderson, R.E., McDonald, C.J., Weiner, M., and Hui, S.L., "How Many Deaths are Due to Medical Errors?," *Journal of American Medical Association*, Vol. 284, No. 17, 2000, pp. 2187–2189.

171. Hupert, N., Lawthers, A.G., Brennan, T.A., and Peterson, L.M., "Processing the Tort Deterrent Signal: a Qualitative Study," *Social Science Medicine*, Vol. 43, No. 1, 1996, pp. 1–11.

172. Hyman, W.A., "Errors in the Use of Medical Equipment," *Human Error in Medicine*, M.S. Bogner, (ed), Lawrence Erlbaum Associates Publishers, Hillsdale, New Jersey, 1994, pp. 327–348.

173. Ibojie, J. and Urbaniak, S.J., "Comparing Near Misses with Actual Mistransfusion Events: a More Accurate Reflection of Transfusion Errors," *British Journal of Haematology*, Vol. 108, 2000, pp. 458–460.

174. *Improving Patient Care by Reporting Problems with Medical Devices*, A MedWatch Education Article, Food and Drug Administration, Rockville, Maryland, September 1997.

175. *Informing the Future: Critical Issues in Health Care Systems*, Institute of Medicine, National Academy Press, Washington, D.C., 2001, pp. 17–23.

176. "Is there a Cure for Drug Errors?," In Editorials, *British Medical Journal*, Vol. 311, 1995, pp. 463–464.

177. Iseli, K.S. and Burger, S., "Diagnostic Errors in Three Medical Eras: A Necropsy Study," *The Lancet*, Vol. 355, 2000, pp. 2027–2031.

178. Ivy, M.E. and Cohn, K., "Human Error in Hospitals and Industrial Accidents," *Journal of the American College of Surgeons*, Vol. 192, No. 3, 2001, p. 421.

179. Jackson, T., "How the Media Report Medical Errors," *British Medical Journal*, Vol. 322, 2001, pp. 562–564.

180. James, B.C. and Hammond, E.H., "The Challenge of Variation in Medical Practice," *Archives of Pathology and Laboratory Medicine*, Vol. 124, No. 7, 2000, pp. 1001–1004.

181. Jameson, F.L., "Exposing Medical Mistakes," *New York Times* , 24 February 2000.

182. Johnson, C., (ed), *Proceedings of the First Workshop on Human Error and Clinical Systems (HECS'99)*, Glasgow Accident Analysis Group Technical Report G99-1, University of Glasgow, Glasgow, UK, 1999.

183. Jones, J. and Hunter D., "Qualitative Research: Consensus Methods for Medical and Health Services Research," *British Medical Journal*, Vol. 311, 1995, pp. 376–380.

184. Joice, P., Hanna, G.B., and Cuschieri, A., "Errors Enacted During Endoscopic Surgery — A Human Reliability Analysis," *Applied Ergonomics*, Vol. 29, No. 6, 1998, pp. 409–415.

185. Kaye, R. and Crowley, J., *Medical Device User-safety: Incorporating Human Factors Engineering into Risk Management*, CDRH, Office of Health and Industry Programs, US Department of Health and Human Services, Washington, D.C., 2000.

186. Keenan, R.L. and Boyan, P., "Cardiac Arrest Due to Anesthesia," *Journal of American Medical Association*, Vol. 253, 1985, pp. 2373–2377.

187. Keller, J.P., "Human Factors Issues in Surgical Devices, *Proceeding of the First Symposium on Human Factors in Medical Devices*, 1989, pp. 34–36.

188. Kieffer, R.G., "Validation and the Human Element," *Pda Journal of Pharmaceutical Science and Technology*, Vol. 52, No. 2, 1998, pp. 52–54.

189. Kirwan, B., "Human Error Identification Techniques for Risk Assessment of High Risk System, Part 1: Review and Evaluation of Techniques," *Applied Ergonomics*, Vol. 29, No. 3, 1998, pp. 157–178.

190. Kirwan, B., "Human Error Identification Techniques for Risk Assessment of High Risk System, Part 2: Towards a Framework Approach," *Applied Ergonomics*, Vol. 29, No. 5, 1998, pp. 299–318.

191. Klemola, U.M., "The Psychology of Human Error Revisited," *European Journal of Anaesthesiology*, Vol. 17, No. 6, 2000, p. 401.

192. Knaus, W.A., Draper, E.A., and Wagner, D.P., "An Evaluation of Outcome from Intensive Care in Major Medical Centres," *Annals of Internal Medicine*, Vol. 104, 1986, pp. 410–418.

193. Kohn, L.T., Corrigan, J.M., and Donaldson, M.S., (eds), *To Err Is Human: Building a Safer Health System*, Institute of Medicine, National Academy Press, Washington, D.C., 1999.

194. Koren, G. and Robert, H.H., "Paediatric Medication Errors: Predicting and Preventing Tenfold Disasters," *Journal of Clinical Pathology*, Vol. 34, 1994, pp. 1043–1045.

195. Kraman, S.S. and Hamm, G., "Risk Management: Extreme Honesty May be the Best Policy," *Annals of Internal Medicine*, Vol. 131, No. 12, 1999, pp. 693–967.

196. Kumar, V., Barcellos, W.A., and Mehta, M.P., "An Analysis of Critical Events in a Teaching Department for Quality Assurance: A Survey of Mishaps During Anesthesia," *Anesthesia*, Vol. 43, No. 10, 1988, pp. 879–883.

197. Kyriacou, D.N. and Coben, J.N., "Errors in Emergency Medicine: Research Strategies," *Academic Emergency Medicine*, Vol. 7, No. 11, 2000, pp. 1201–1203.

198. Laura, L., "Human Error in Patient Controlled Analgesia: Incident Reports and Experimental Evaluation," *Proceedings of the Human Factors and Ergonomics Society*, Vol. 2, 1998, pp. 1043–1047.

199. Le Cocq, A.D., "Application of Human Factors Engineering in Medical Product Design," *Journal of Clinical Engineering*, Vol. 12, No. 4, 1987, pp. 271–277.

200. Leape L.L., Gullen, D.J., and Clapps, M.D., "Pharmacist Participation on Physician Rounds and Adverse Drug Events in the Intensive Care Unit," *Journal of American Medical Association*, Vol. 282, No. 3, 1999, pp. 267–270.

201. Leape, L.L, Woods, D.D., Hatlie, M.J., and Kizre, K.W., "Promoting Patient Safety by Preventing Medical Error," *Journal of American Medical Association*, Vol. 280, No. 16, 1998, pp. 1444–1448.

202. Leape, L.L., Kabcenell, A.I., Gandhi, T.K., Carver, P., Nolan, T.W., and Berwick, D.M., "Reducing Adverse Drug Events: Lessons From a Breakthrough Series Collaborative," *Joint Commission Journal on Quality Improvement*, Vol. 26, No. 6, 2000, pp. 321–331.

203. Leape, L.L., Swankin, D.S., and Yessian, M.R., "A Conversation On Medical Injury," *Public Health Reports*, Vol. 114, 1999, pp. 302–317.

204. Leape, L.L., "The Preventability of Medical Injury," *Human Error in Medicine*, Bogner M.S., (ed), Lawrence Erlbaum Associates Publishers, Hillsdale, New Jersey, 1994, pp. 13–27.

205. Leape, L.L., "Error in Medicine," *Journal of American Medical Association*, Vol. 272, No. 23, 1994, pp. 1851–1857.

206. Leape, L.L., Cullen, D.J., Laird, N., Petersen, L.A., Teich, J.M., Burdick, E., Hickey, M., Kleefield, S., Shea, B., Vander Vliet, M., and Seger, D.L., "Effect of Computerized Physician Order Entry and a Team Intervention on Prevention of Serious Medication Errors," *Journal of American Medical Association*, Vol. 280, No. 15, 1998, pp. 1311–1316.

207. Liang, B.A., "Error in Medicine: Legal Impediments to US Reform," *Journal of Health Politics, Policy and Law*, Vol. 24, No. 1, 1999, pp. 28–58.

208. Ludbrook, G.L., Webb, R.K., and Fox, M.A., "The Australian Incident Monitoring Study: Physical Injuries and Environmental Safety in Anaesthesia: An Analysis of 2000 Incident reports," *Anaesthesia and Intensive Care*, Vol. 21, No. 5, 1993, pp. 659–663.

209. Lori, A.B. and Carol, S., "An Alternative Strategy for Studying Adverse Events in Medical Care," *Lancet*, Vol. 349, 1997, pp. 309–313.

210. Ludbrook, G.L., Webb, R.K., Fox, M.A., and Singletons, R.J., "Problems Before Induction of Anaesthesia: An Analysis of 2000 Incidents Report," *Anaesthesia and Intensive Care*, Vol. 21, 1993, pp. 593–595.

211. Lunn, J. and Devlin, H., "Lessons From the Confidential Inquiry into Preoperative Deaths in Three NHS Regions," *Lancet*, Vol. 2, 1987, pp. 1384–1386.

212. Maddox, M.E., "Designing Medical Devices to Minimize Human Error," *Medical Device Diagnostic Industry Magazine*, Vol. 19, No. 5, 1997, pp. 160–180.

213. *Making Health Care Safer: A Critical Analysis of Patient Safety Practices*, Agency for Healthcare Research and Quality, Rockville, Maryland, U.S.A., 1998.

214. "Managing the Risks from Medical Product Use," *Report to the FDA Commissioner from The Task Force on Risk Management*, US Department of Health and Human Services, Food and Drug Administration, Washington, D.C., USA, May 1999.

215. Marconi, M. and Sirchia, G., "Increasing Transfusion Safety by Reducing Human Error," *Current Opinion in Haematology*, Vol. 7, No. 6, 2000, pp. 382–386.

216. Marsden, P. and Hollnagel, E., "Human Interaction with Technology: the Accidental User," *Acta Psychologica*, Vol. 91, No. 3, 1996, pp. 345–358.

217. Mayor, S., "English NHS to set up New Reporting System for Errors," *British Medical Journal*, Vol. 320, 2000, p. 1689.

218. McCadden, P., "Medical Errors," *Proceedings of a Conference on Enhancing Patient Safety and Reducing Errors in Health Care*, National Patient Safety Foundation, Rancho Mirage, Chicago, 1999, pp. 68–69.

219. McClure, M.L., "Human Error — A Professional Dilemma, *Journal of Professional Nursing*, Vol. 7, No. 4, 1991, p. 207.

220. McConnel, E.A., "Pointed Strategies for Needle Stick Prevention," *Nursing Management*, Vol. 30, No. 1, 1999, pp. 57–60.

221. McCray, S., *Medical Errors in the US Medical System*, Institute of Medicine, National Academy of Medicine, National Academy Press, Washington, DC, USA, 1999.

222. McDonald, J.S. and Peterson, S., "Lethal Errors in Anaesthesiology," *Anaesthesiology*, Vol. 63, 1985, p. A497.

223. McManus, B., "A Move to Electronic Patient Records in the Community: a Qualitative Case Study of a Clinical Data Collection System, Problems Caused by Inattention to Users and Human Error," *Topics in Health Information Management*, Vol. 20, No. 4, 2000, pp. 23–37.

224. McManus, J., "Hong Kong Issues Guidelines to Prevent Further Medical Blunders," *British Medical Journal*, Vol. 315, 1997, pp. 967–972.

225. *Medical Errors: The Scope of the Problem*, Agency for Healthcare Research and Quality, Food and Drug Administration, Rockville, Maryland, 2000.

226. Mehra, R.H. and Eagle, K.A., "Missed Diagnosis of Acute Coronary Syndromes in the Emergency Room — Continuing Challenges," *New England Journal of Medicine*, Vol. 342, No. 16, 2000, pp. 1207–1209.

227. Meyboom, R.H., Lindquist, M., Stahl, M., Bate, A., and Edwards, I.R., "A Retrospective Evaluation of a Data Mining Approach to Aid Finding New Adverse Drug Reaction Signals in the WHO International Database," *Drug Safety*, Vol. 23, No. 6, 2000, pp. 533–542.

228. Michael P., "Congress Backs Away from Mandatory Reporting of Medical Errors," *Medical Economics*, Vol. 77, No. 16, 2000, pp. 25–26.

229. Moeller, J., O'Reilly, J.B., and Elser, J., "Quality Management in German Health Care — The EFQM Excellence Model," *International Journal of Health Care Quality Assurance*, Vol. 13, No. 6, 2000, pp. 254–258.

230. Moliver, M., "Computerization Helps Reduce Human Error in Patient Dosing," *Contemporary Longterm Care*, Vol. 10, No. 10, 1987, pp. 56–58.

231. Moray, D., "Error Reduction as a Systems Problem," *Human Error in Medicine*, Bogner, M.S., (ed), Lawrence Erlbaum Associates Publishers, Hillsdale, New Jersey, 1994, pp. 67–92.

232. Morris, G.P. and Morris, R.W., "Anaesthesia and Fatigue: an Analysis of the First 10 Years of the Australian Incident Monitoring Study 1987–1997," *Anaesthesia and Intensive Care*, Vol. 28, No. 3, 2000, pp. 300–304.

233. Moyer, P., "Medical Mistakes are Leading Cause of Death and Disability," *WebMD Medical News*, November, 1999.

234. Nakata, Y., Fujiwara, M.O., and Goto, T., "Risk Attitudes of Anesthesiologists and Surgeons in Clinical Decision Making with Expected Years of Life," *Journal of Clinical Anesthesia*, Vol. 12, 2000, pp. 146–150.

235. Narumi, J., "Analysis of Human Error in Nursing Care," *Accident Analysis and Prevention*, Vol. 31, 1999, pp. 625–629.

236. Naylor, D., "Reporting Medical Mistakes and Misconduct," *Canadian Medical Association Journal*, Vol. 160, No. 9, 1999, pp. 1323–1324.

237. Newbower, R.S., Cooper, J.B., and Lon, C.D., "Failure Analysis — Human Element," *Essential Noninvasive Monitoring In Anaesthesia*, Gravenstein, J.S., Ronald, S.N., Allen, K. Ream, N. Ty, S., and John, B., (eds), Grune & Stratton Publishers, New York, NY, 1980, pp. 269–282.

238. Newhall, C., "The Institute of Medicine Report on Medical Errors," *The New England Journal of Medicine*, Vol. 343, No. 9, 2000, pp. 105–109.

239. Nobel, J.L., Medical Device Failures and Adverse Effects, *Pediatric Emergency Care*, Vol. 7, 1991, pp. 120–123.

240. Nolan, T.W., "System Changes to Improve Patient Safety," *British Medical Journal*, Vol. 320, 2000, pp. 771–773.

241. Nordenberg, T., "Make No Mistakes: Medical Errors can be Deadly Serious," *FDA Consumer Magazine*, September–October 2000, pp. 104–106.

242. O'Leary, D.S., "Accreditation's Role in Reducing Medical Errors," *British Medical Journal*, Vol. 320, 2000, pp. 727–728.

243. O'Rourke, K., "The Human Factors in Medical Error," *New England Journal of Medicine*, Vol. 304, No. 11, 1981, pp. 634–641.

244. O'Shea, A., "Factors Contributing to Medication Errors: A Literature Review," *Journal of Clinical Nursing*, Vol. 8, 1999, pp. 496–504.

245. Ovretveit, J., "System Negligence is at the Root of Medical Error," *International Journal of Health Care Quality Assurance*, Vol. 13, No. 3, 2000, pp. 103–105.

246. Passey, R.D., "Foresight Begins with FMEA, Delivering Accurate Risk Assessments," *Medical Device Technology*, Vol. 10, No. 2, 1999, pp. 88–92.

247. Phillips, D.P., Christenfeld, N., and Glynn, L.M., "Increase in US Medication-error Deaths Between 1983–1993," *Lancet*, Vol. 1351, 1998, pp. 1024–1029.

248. Pietro, D.A., Shyavitz, L.J., Smith, R.A., and Auerbach, B.S., "Detecting and Reporting Medical Errors: Why the Dilemma?," *British Medical Journal*, Vol. 320, 2000, pp. 794–796.

249. Podell, R.N. and Smith, W.P., "When our Doctor Doesn't Know Best: Medical Mistakes Even the Best Doctors Make — and how to Protect Yourself," *Publishers Weekly*, Vol. 241, No. 49, 1994, p. 75.

250. Peters, M., "Implementation of Rules-based Computerized Bedside Prescribing and Administration: Intervention Study," *British Medical Journal*, Vol. 320, 2000, pp. 750–753.

251. Posner, K.L. and Freund, P.R., "Trends in Quality of Anaesthesia Care Associated with Changing Staffing Patterns, Productivity and Concurrency of Case Supervision in a Teaching Hospital," *Anaesthesiology*, Vol. 91, No. 3, 1999, pp. 839–847.

252. Preboth, M., "Medication Errors in Paediatric Patients," *American Family Physician*, Vol. 63, No. 2, 2001, p. 678.

253. Purday, J.P., "Monitoring During Paediatric Cardiac Anaesthesia," *Canadian Journal of Anaesthesia*, Vol. 41, No. 9, 1994, pp. 818–844.

254. Rachlin, J.A., "Human Factors and Medical Devices," *FDA USER Facility Reporting, A Quarterly Bulletin to Assist Hospitals, Nursing Homes, and Other Device User Facilities*, No. 12, Summer 1995, pp. 86–89.

255. Rao, S.N., "Errors in the Treatment of Tuberculosis in Baltimore," *Journal of American Medical Association*, Vol. 283, No. 19, 2000, p. 2502.

256. Rasmussen, J., "Human Error and the Problem of Causality in Analysis of Accidents," *Philosophical Transactions of the Royal Society of London-Series B: Biological Sciences*, Vol. 327, No. 1241, 1990, pp. 449–460.

257. Rascona, D., Gubler, K.D., Kobus, D.A., Amundson, D., and Moses, J.D., "A Computerized Medical Incident Reporting System for Errors in the Intensive Care Unit: Initial Evaluation of Interrater Agreement," *Military Medicine*, Vol. 166, No. 4, 2001, pp. 350–353.

258. Reason, J., "Human Error: Models and Management," *British Medical Journal*, Vol. 320, 2000, pp. 768–770.

259. Reed, L., Blegen, M.A., and Goode, C.S., "Adverse Patient Occurrences as a Measure of Nursing Care Quality," *Journal of Nursing Administration*, Vol. 28, 1998, pp. 62–69.

260. "Reducing Errors, Improving Safety," *Letters, British Medical Journal*, Vol. 321, 2000, pp. 505–509.
261. Rendell-Baker, L., "Some Gas Machine Hazards and Their Elimination," *Anaesthesia Analgesia*, Vol. 88, No. 1, 1977, pp. 26–33.
262. Richard, C. and Woods, C., *Operating at the Sharp Ends: the Complexity of Human Error*, Bogner, M.S., (ed), Human Error in Medicine, Hillsdale, NJ, Lawrence Erlbaum Associates, 1994, pp. 255–310.
263. Richard, J., "Identifying Ways to Reduce Surgical Errors," *Journal of American Medical Association*, Vol. 275, No. 1, 1996, p. 35.
264. Richard, K., "Prescription Errors Tied to Lack of Advice: Pharmacists Skirting Law, Massachusetts Study Finds," *Boston Globe*, 10 February, 1999, Metro, B1.
265. Richards, C.F. and Cannon, C.P., "Reducing Medication Errors: Potential Benefits of Bolus Thrombolytic Agents," *Academic Emergency Medicine*, Vol. 7, No. 11, 2000, pp. 1285–1289.
266. Richards, P., Kennedy, I.M., and Woolf, L., "Managing Medical Mishaps," *British Medical Journal*, Vol. 313, 1996, pp. 243–244.
267. Ritchie, J., "Doctors Make Mistakes that are Less Obvious than Lawyers' Mistakes," *British Medical Journal*, Vol. 310, 1995, pp. 1671–1672.
268. Robert, D.W. and Robert, B.H., "Preventable Deaths: Who, How Often, and Why?," *Annals of Internal Medicine*, Vol. 109, 1998, pp. 582–589.
269. Rogers, A.S., Isreal, E., and Smith, C.R., "A Physician Knowledge, Attitudes, and Behaviour Related to Reporting Adverse Drug Events," *Archives of Internal Medicine*, Vol. 148, 1988, pp. 1596–1600.
270. Roelofse J.A. and Shipton E.A., "Obstruction of a Breathing Circuit: a Case Study," *South African Medical Journal*, Vol. 66, No. 13, 1984, pp. 501–502.
271. Rosenthal, M.M. and Lloyd, S.B., (ed), *Medical Mishaps: Pieces of the Puzzle*, Open University Press, London, 1999.
272. Rovner, J., "Washington Wakes up to Medical Errors," *Business & Health*, January 2000, p. 19.
273. Rubin, S.B. and Zoloth, L., "Margin of Error: The Ethics of Mistakes in the Practice of Medicine," *The New England Journal of Medicine*, Vol. 344, No. 5, 2001, pp. 374–376.
274. Rudov, M.H., "Professional Standards Review in Health Systems," in *Human Factors in Health Care*, Pickett, R.M. and Triggs, T.J., (ed), Lexington Books, Lexington, Massachusetts, 1977, pp. 7–47.
275. Runciman, W.B., Sellen, A., Webb, R.K., Williamson, J.A., and Current, M., "Errors, Incidents and Accidents in Anaesthetic Practice," *Anaesthesia and Intensive Care*, Vol. 21, No. 5, 1993, pp. 506–519.
276. Runciman, W.B., Webb, R.K., and Lee, R., "System Failure: An Analysis of 2000 Incidents Reports," *Anaesthesia and Intensive Care*, Vol. 21, No. 5, 1993, pp. 684–695.
277. Runciman, W.B., Helps, S.C., Sexton, E.J., and Malpass, A., "A Classification for Incidents and Accidents in the Health-Care System," *Journal of Quality and Clinical Practice*, Vol. 18/3, 1998, pp. 199–212.

278. Russell, C., "Human Error: Avoidable Mistakes Kill 100000 a Year," *The Washington Post*, February, 1992, p. WH 7.

279. Sacchetti, A., Sacchetti, C., Carraccio, C., and Gerardi, M., "The Potential for Errors in Children with Special Health Care Needs," *Academic Emergency Medicine*, Vol. 7, No. 11, 2000, pp. 1330–1333.

280. Sawyer, D., *Do it by Design: an Introduction to Human Factors in Medical Devices*, CDRH, US Department of Health and Human Services, Food and Drug Administration, Washington, D.C., 2000.

281. Scheffler, A.L. and Zipperer, L., "Patient Safety," *Proceedings of the Symposium on the Enhancing Patient Safety and Reducing Errors in Health Care*, Rancho Mirage, California, November 1998, pp. 115–120.

282. Scott, J.S., "To Err Is Human: To Forgive, Un-American," *Healthcare Financial Management*, February 2000, pp. 26–27.

283. Scott, D., "Preventing Medical Mistakes," *RN Magazine*, Vol. 63, No. 8, 2000, pp. 60–64.

284. Shannon, L., "X-rays and Human Error," *Australian Family Physician*, Vol. 15, No. 11, 1986, p. 1455.

285. Senders, J. and Moray, N., *Human Error: Cause, Prediction, and Reduction*, Lawrence Erlbaum Associates, Hillsdale, New Jersey, 1991.

286. Senders, J.W., "Medical Devices, Medical Errors, and Medical Accidents," *Human Error in Medicine*, Bogner, M.S., (ed), Lawrence Erlbaum Associates Publishers, Hillsdale, New Jersey, 1994, pp. 159–177.

287. Sexton, J.B., Thomas, E.J., and Helmreich, R.L., "Error, Stress, and Teamwork in Medicine and Aviation: Cross Sectional Surveys," *British Medical Journal*, Vol. 320, 2000, pp. 745–749.

288. Shanghnessy, A.F. and Nickel, R.O., "Prescription-writing Patterns and Errors in a Family Medicine Residency Program," *Journal of Family Practice*, Vol. 29, No. 3, 1989, pp. 290–296.

289. Shapiro, J.P., "Taking the Mistakes Out of Medicine," *US News and World Report*, Vol. 129, No. 3, 2000, pp. 50–54.

290. Shea, C.E. and Battles, J.B., "A System of Analyzing Medical Errors to Improve GME Eurricula and Programs," *Academic Medicine*, Vol. 76, No. 2, 2001, pp. 125–133.

291. Shelton, N., "To Err is Human," *Skeptical Inquirer*, Vol. 20, No. 3, 1996, pp. 21–22.

292. Sheridan, T.B. and Thompson J.M., "People Versus Computers in Medicine," *Human Error in Medicine*, Bogner M.S., (ed), Lawrence Erlbaum Associates Publishers, Hillsdale, New Jersey, 1994, pp. 141–159.

293. Shinn, J.A., "Root Cause Analysis: a Method of Addressing Errors and Patient Risk," *Progress in Cardiovascular Nursing*, Vol. 15, No. 1, 2000, p. 25.

294. Short, T.G., O'Regan, A., and Jayasuriya, J.P., "Improvements in Anesthetic Care Resulting from a Critical Incident Reporting Programme," *Anaesthesia*, Vol. 57, No. 7, 1996, pp. 615–621.

295. Short, T.G., O'Regan, A., and Oh, T.E., "Critical Incident Reporting in an Anaesthetic Department Assurance Programme," *Anaesthesia*, Vol. 47, 1992. pp. 3–7.

296. Smith, D.L., "Medication Errors and DTC Ads," *Pharmaceutical Executive*, February 2000, p. 129.

297. Smith, J., "Study into Medical errors Planned for the UK," *British Medical Journal*, Vol. 319, 1999, pp. 1091–1092.

298. Souhrada, L., "Abbott Infuses I.V. Business with Growth," *Hospitals*, Vol. 64, No. 1, 1990, p. 67.

299. Souhrada, L., "Human Error Limits MRI'S Quality Potential," *Hospitals*, Vol. 63, No. 10, 1989, p. 38.

300. Souhrada, L., "Man Meets Machine: Buying Right can Reduce Human Error," *Materials Management in Health Care*, Vol. 4, No. 11, 1995, pp. 20–22.

301. Spath, P.L., "Medical Errors: Root Cause Analysis," *OR Manager*, Vol. 14, No. 9, 1998, pp. 40–41.

302. Spencer, F.C., "Human Error in Hospitals and Industrial Accidents: Current Concepts," *Journal of the American College of Surgeons*, Vol. 191, No. 4, 2000, pp. 410–418.

303. Spice, C., "Misdiagnosis of Ventricular Tachycardia," *The Lancet*, Vol. 354, 1999, pp. 2165–2169.

304. Staender, S., Davies, J., Helmreich, B., Sexton, B., and Kaufmann, M., "The Anaesthesia Critical Incident Reporting System: an Experience-based Database," *International Journal of Medical Informatics*, Vol. 47, 1997, pp. 87–90.

305. Stahlhut, R.W., Gosbee, J.W., and Gardner-Bonneau, D.J., "A Human-centered Approach to Medical Informatics for Medical Students, Residents, and Practicing Clinicians," *Academic Medicine*, Vol. 72, No. 10, 1997, pp. 881–887.

306. Stanton, N.A. and Stevenage, S.V., "Learning to Predict Human Error: Issues of Acceptability, Reliability and Validity," *Ergonomics*, Vol. 41, No. 11, 1998, pp. 1737–1756.

307. Stewart, M.J., "Toxic Risks of Inappropriate Therapy," *Clinical Biochemistry*, Vol. 23, 1990, pp. 73–77.

308. Stump, L.S., "Re-engineering the Medication Error-reporting Process: Removing the Blame and improving the System," *American Journal of Health-System Pharmacy*, Vol. 57, Suppl. 4, 2000, pp. S10–17.

309. Taylor, G., "What is Minimal Monitoring," *Essential Non-invasive Monitoring In Anaesthesia*, Gravenstein, J.S., Newbower, R.S., Ream, A.K., Smith, N.T., and Barden, J., (eds), Grune and Stratton Publishers, New York, NY, 1980, pp. 263–267.

310. Tarcinale, M.A., "Patient Classification: Cutting the Margin of Human Error," *Nursing Management*, Vol. 17, No. 10, 1986, pp. 49–51.

311. Thierry, G., Dhainaut, J.F., Joseph, T., and Journois, D., "Iatrogenic Complications in Adult Intensive Care Units: a Prospective Two-center Study," *Critical Care Medicine*, Vol. 21, No. 1, 1993, pp. 40–52.

312. Thomas, E. J. and Brennan, T.A., "Incidence and Types of Preventable Adverse Events in Elderly Patients: Population-based Review of Medical Records," *British Medical Journal*, Vol. 320, 2000, pp. 741–744.

313. Thomas, E.J., Studdert, D.M., and Newhouse, J.P., "Costs of Medical Injuries in Utah and Colorado," *Inquiry*, Vol. 36, 1999, pp. 255–265.

314. Thomas, E.J., Studdert, D.M., and Burstin, H. R., "Incidence of Adverse Events due to Medical Error in the US," *Medical Care*, Vol. 38, No. 3, 2000, pp. 261–271.

315. Thomas, E.J., Sherwood, G.D., and Adams-McNeill, J., "Identifying and Addressing Medical Errors in Pain Mismanagement," *Joint Commission Journal on Quality Improvement*, Vol. 27, No. 4, 2001, pp. 191–199.

316. Thomas, E.J., Studdert, D.M., Runciman, W.B., Webb, R.K., Sexton, E.J., Wilson, R.M., Gibberd, R.W., Harrison, B.T., and Brennan, T.A., "A Comparison of Iatrogenic Injury Studies in Australia and the USA, I: Context, Methods, Casemix, Population, Patient and Hospital Characteristics," *International Journal for Quality in Health Care*, Vol. 12, No. 5, 2000, pp. 371–378.

317. Van Grunsven, P.R., "Criminal Prosecution of Health Care Providers for Clinical Mistakes and Fatal Errors: Is Bad Medicine a Crime?," *Journal of Health and Hospital Law*, Vol. 29, 1996, p. 107.

318. Varricchio, F., "Another Type of Medication Error," *Southern Medical Journal*, Vol. 93, No. 8, 2000, p. 834.

319. Vickers, M.D., "The Psychology of Human Error," *European Journal of Anesthesiology*, Vol. 16, No. 8, 1999, p. 578.

320. Vincent, C.A., "Research into Medical Accidents: a Case of Negligence?," *British Medical Journal*, Vol. 299, 1989, pp. 1150–1153.

321. Vincent, C., Neale, G., and Woloshynowych, M., "Adverse Events in British Hospitals: Preliminary Retrospective Record Review," *British Medical Journal*, Vol. 322, 2001, pp. 517–519.

322. Vincent, C., Taylor, S., and Chapman J.E., "How to Investigate and Analyze Clinical Incidents: Clinical Risk Unit and Association of Litigation and Risk Management Protocol," *British Medical Journal*, Vol. 320, 2000, pp. 777–778.

323. Wallace, D.R. and Kuhn, R.D., "Lessons from 342 Medical Device Failures," in *Information Technology Laboratory, National Institute of Standards and Technology*, Gaithersburg, Maryland, USA, 2000, pp. 25–31.

324. Wears, R.L., Janiak, B., Moorhead, J.C., Kellermann, A.L., Yeh, C.S., Rice, M.M., Jay, G., Perry, S.J., and Woolard, R., "Human Error in Medicine: Promise and Pitfalls, Part 1," *Annals of Emergency Medicine*, Vol. 36, No. 1, 2000, pp. 58–60.

325. Wears, R.L., Janiak, B., Moorhead, J.C., Kellermann, A.L., Yeh, C.S., Rice, M.M., Jay, G., Perry, S.J., and Woolard, R., "Human Error in Medicine: Promise and Pitfalls, Part 2," *Annals of Emergency Medicine*, Vol. 36, No. 2, 2000, pp. 142–144.

326. Wears, R.L. and Leape L.L., "Human Error in Emergency Medicine," *Annals of Emergency Medicine*, Vol. 34, 1999, pp. 370–372.

327. Webb, R.K., Russell, W.J., and Klepper, I., "Equipment Failure: an Analysis of 2000 Incidents Reports," *Anaesthesia and Intensive Care*, Vol. 21, No. 5, 1993, pp. 673–677.

328. Welch, D.L., "Human Factors in the Health Care Facility," *Biomedical Instrumentation and Technology*, Vol. 32, No. 3, 1998, pp. 311–316.

329. Webster, S.A., "Technology Helps Reduce Mistakes on Medications," *The Detroit News*, February, 2000.

330. Wechsler, J., "Manufacturers Challenged to Reduce Medication Errors," *Pharmaceutical Technology*, February 2000, pp. 14–22.

331. Weilgart, S.N., Ship, A.N., and Aronson, M.D., "Confidential Clinican-reported Surveillance of Adverse Events Among Medical Inpatients," *Journal General Internal Medicine*, Vol. 15, 2000, pp. 470–477.

332. Weingart, S.N., Wilkson, R.S., and Gibberd, R.W., "Epidemiology of Medical Error," *British Medical Journal*, Vol. 320, 2000, pp. 774–776.

333. Weinger, M.B., "Anesthesia Equipment and Human Error," *Journal of Clinical Monitoring and Computing*, Vol. 15, No. 5, 1999, pp. 319–323.

334. Welch, D.L., "Human Error and Human Factors Engineering in Health Care," *Biomedical Instrumentation and Technology*, Vol. 31, No. 6, 1997, pp. 627–631.

335. Welch, D.L., "Human Factors Analysis and Design Support in Medical Device Development," *Biomedical Instrumentation and Technology*, Vol. 32, No. 1, 1998, pp. 77–82.

336. Wenz, B. and Mercuriali, F., "Practical Methods to Improve Transfusion Safety by Using Novel Blood Unit and Patient Identification Systems," *Pathology Patterns*, Vol. 107, No. 4, 2000, pp. S12–16.

337. Widman, L.E. and Tong, D.A., "EINTHOVEN and Tolerance for Human Error: Design Issues in Decision Support System for Cardiac Arrhythmia Interpretation," *Proceedings of the AMIA Annual Fall Symposium*, 1986, pp. 224–228.

338. Wikland, M.E., *Medical Device and Equipment Design*, Interpharm Press Inc., Buffalo Grove, Illinois, 1995.

339. Wiklund, M.E., Weinger, M.B., Pantiskas, C., and Carstensen, P., "Incorporating Human Factors into the Design of Medical Devices," *JAMA*, Vol. 280, No. 17, 1998, p. 1484.

340. Williamson, J.A., Webb, R.K., and Sellen, A., "Human Failure: an Analysis of 2000 Incidents Reports," *Anaesthsia and Intensive Care*, Vol. 21, No. 5, 1993, pp. 678–683.

341. Willis, G., "Failure Modes and Effects Analysis in Clinical Engineering," *Journal of Clinical Engineering*, Vol. 17, No. 1, 1992, pp. 59–63.

342. Wright, D., *Critical Incident Reporting in an Intensive Care Unit: 10 Years' Experience*, Intensive Therapy Unit, Western General Hospital, Edinburgh, Scotland, 1999.

343. Woods, D.D. and Hollnagel, E., "Cognitive Systems Engineering: New Wine in New Bottles," *International Journal of Human-computer Studies*, Vol. 51, No. 2, 1999, pp. 339–356.

344. Wu, A.W., Folkman, S., and McPhee, S.J., "How House Officers Cope with Their Mistakes," *Western Journal of Medicine*, Vol. 159, 1993, pp. 565–569.

345. Wu, A.W., Folkman, S., and McPhee, S.J., "Do House Officers Learn From Their Mistakes," *Journal of American Medical Association*, Vol. 265, No. 16, 1991, pp. 2089–2094.

346. Wu, A.W., "Handling Hospital Errors: Is Disclosure the Best defence?," *Annuls of Internal Medicine*, Vol. 131, No. 12, 1999, pp. 970–972.
347. Wu, A.W., "Medical Error: The Second Victim," *British Medical Journal*, Vol. 320, 2000, pp. 726–727.
348. Wyant, G.M., *Mechanical Misadventures of Anaesthesia*, University of Toronto Press, Toronto, 1978.
349. Zimmerman, J.E., Knaus, W.A., Wagner, D.P., Draper, E.A., and Lawrence, D.E., "The Range of Intensive Care Services Today," *Journal of American Medical Association*, Vol. 246, No. 23, 1981, pp. 2711–2716.
350. Zimmerman, J.E., Shortell, S.M., Rousseau, D.M., Duffy, J., and Gillies, R.R., "Improving Intensive Care: Observations Based on Organizational Case Studies in Nine Intensive Care Units: A Prospective Multicenter Study," *Critical Care Medicine*, Vol. 21, No. 10, 1983, pp. 1443–1451.

Index